When the Belly Button Pops, the Baby's Done

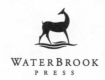

A Month-by-Month Guide to Surviving (and Loving) Your Pregnancy

■ ■ ■

LORILEE CRAKER

WATERBROOK
PRESS

WHEN THE BELLY BUTTON POPS, THE BABY'S DONE
PUBLISHED BY WATERBROOK PRESS
2375 Telstar Drive, Suite 160
Colorado Springs, Colorado 80920
A division of Random House, Inc.

The author of this book is not a physician, and the ideas, procedures, and suggestions in this book are not intended as a substitute for the medical advice of a trained health professional. All matters regarding your health require medical supervision. Consult your physician before adopting the suggestions in this book, as well as about any condition that may require diagnosis or medical attention. The author and publisher disclaim any liability arising directly or indirectly from the use of the book.

All Scripture quotations, unless otherwise indicated, are taken from the *Holy Bible, New International Version*®. NIV®. Copyright © 1973, 1978, 1984 by International Bible Society. Used by permission of Zondervan Publishing House. All rights reserved. Scripture quotations marked (KJV) are taken from the *King James Version*.

ISBN 1-57856-486-7

Library of Congress Cataloging-in-Publication Data
Craker, Lorilee.

  When the belly button pops, the baby's done : a month-by-month guide to surviving (and loving) your pregnancy / Lorilee Craker.— 1st ed.
      p. cm.
  ISBN 1-57856-486-7
  1. Pregnancy—Popular works. 2. Childbirth—Popular works. I. Title.

RG525 .C815 2002
618.2—dc21

                                                              2002011150

Printed in the United States of America
2004

10 9 8 7 6 5 4

Contents

Preface

I had the opportunity and pleasure of reading Lorilee's book during my pregnancy, and the information regarding physical, mental, emotional, social, and spiritual issues is right on target. Many times I stopped to say to myself, "Wow, this is exactly how I feel, and this is also exactly what I need to hear to know how to deal with this." I had read other pregnancy information that just depressed me by causing me to dread all the negative things I might experience, but Lorilee's book is different: It tells it like it is, yet gives you hope, understanding, and strategies to deal with the less-than-pleasant aspects of pregnancy.

A survey of recent medical literature reveals a trend in research showing how our spirituality is connected to our health. This concept is nicely incorporated into this book, especially as it describes a time in life that is so emotional and that involves the health of both mother and baby.

This book also celebrates the wonders and joy of it all in a way that makes you realize how awesome it is to be pregnant. All of this, and in an easy-to-read, "I can't put this book down" style!

—Juanita Moses, M.D.
November 2001

Dedication and Acknowledgments

To my mom, Linda Reimer,
because even though you never carried me inside your body,
I was truly born in your heart.

It's been said over and over that writing a book is like being pregnant. Certain individuals have been my "book doulas" all along the way, even in the preconception stage. Therefore my heartfelt gratitude goes out to the following people:

- Linda Holland, for nurturing my writing and my aspirations for so long and for listening ever so well.
- Twila Bennett, my dear friend, for being excited for me and for all your great ideas and fun lunches.
- Dwight Baker, for being a friend as well as former boss and for guiding this novice through some of the tricky aspects of the book business.
- Holly Westenbroek, Leanne Lozada, Sheri Rodriguez, Dawn Uitvlugt, and Grace Miguel for being friends and caregivers to my Jo Jo while I worked on this book. I couldn't have written a decent word if I didn't feel confident that he was in the best of hands.
- "Grandma Pat" Vanderlaan, for scrumptious home-cooked meals, the most loving babysitting, and your perpetual interest in my projects! (That goes for "Grandpa George" too.)
- Cal Haines, for being the first to tell me he thought I had a real shot at making my living by writing (or something to that effect)!

- Bonnie Anderson, Nancy Rubin, Carla Klassen, Lisa Friere, Stephanie Nelson, Becky Wertz Walker, Rachel Vanderlaan, and Mary Jo Haab: My precious sisterhood of pals, channels of grace each one.
- My parents, Abe and Linda Reimer, and my in-laws, Ken and Linda Craker, the Connells, the Bushes, and the Reimers: Your support means everything!
- Lisa Tawn Bergren: I could really start gushing here, but there's just no space! For being an amazing role model, encourager, and friend—and for thinking I should be published—I can never thank you enough.
- Erin Healy, for taking the baton from Lisa with such ease and grace, for your savvy editing brain, and for being so unswervingly supportive, kind, and uplifting!
- And especially for my guys at home, who cheered for me and let me sit in the basement night after night, weekend after weekend, shaping and forming this book. I love you so much!

Introduction

The other day while walking through JCPenney, I spotted the most adorable maternity dress. Suddenly I felt kind of sad, wistful that I probably wouldn't be wearing maternity clothes again. My mind flashed back to last summer, when I was a few months pregnant with my second child, Ezra, and when I started writing this, my second book. I could feel my baby fluttering already, and having survived a rather green-around-the-gills first trimester, I found the second to be pretty much cake. Okay, so I was getting bigger faster than I did when I was pregnant with my first-born, Jonah, and I gave the family basset hound stiff competition in the "Best Waddle" category. True, I was forced to forgo Starbucks (at least the real juice), and my shoes weren't fitting so great. But I was carrying my baby with me, everywhere. We were a pair, inextricably wound up in each other, as close as close can be.

I miss that.

There's nothing like the intense, wonder-filled journey of pregnancy that starts with the anxious scan of an EPT stick and ends in motherhood, with much agony and ecstasy in between. I love pregnancy. Mostly I love it in other people, but I do adore the whole topic! Even the agony part. (For me, the agony kicked in as my huge belly grew and just sat on a crack in my pelvis, the result of an earlier car accident. As I recall, even rolling over in bed caused a wince and an alarming clicking sound, which gets louder and more ominous every time I tell the story. But let's not focus on agony just yet.)

I set out to write this book because I wanted to poke a bit of fun at this miraculous yet utterly ludicrous time in a woman's life when she might be found eating chalk, crying at diaper commercials, and performing discreet vaginal toning exercises—all at once!

At the same time, I recognize that pregnancy isn't all belly laughs. It can also be fearful, unsettling, and stone-cold serious stuff. And so I wanted to write a book on pregnancy that spoke to the whole pregnant person (that would be you), from the top of her pregnantly paranoid brain to the tips of her pregnantly puffy feet. I'm no medical authority—let's agree right now that you will use *What to Expect When You're Expecting* and your doctor for that type of thing—but after two babies, a kabillion hours of research, and oodles of interviews, I'm confident that I've gathered some pretty solid advice for you.

Within these pages are some amazing stories and anecdotes from pregnant pals, past and present, from all over the U.S. and Canada. Their voices shine as they tell about the peerless pregnancy experiences they've had.

One more thing. There's quite a bit of material here on relationships because I think pregnancy is a pivotal time of growing closer to, or farther apart from, the ones we love, including God Himself. The best thing you can do for your baby is to get tight—real tight—with his earthbound dad and his heavenly one. Hopefully the ideas and stories in these pages will set you on the right path to doing just that.

So you're pregnant, huh? How absolutely fabulous! You may throw up in Target, gain a shoe size, and wear a muumuu to the beach, but when you hold your little one in your arms, I promise you, you won't care about any of that.

The Mattress Mambo
and Other Delicate Subjects

This is it, the moment you've waited for—maybe for your entire life. You and your mate have decided to become parents: Ma and Pa. The folks. Matriarch and patriarch of a tribe all your own. Some miniscule sperm and egg might not even know it yet, but they are headed for a close encounter so fraught with Divine Design that no parties involved will ever be the same.

Now it's time for execution, the *doing* phase, the fun part. (Well, one of the fun parts!) I need not say that this is no time to beg off the act of marital love. Who cares if you have a headache, a backache, allergies, or mad cow disease? It's time to get busy! When the next yahoo so subtly inquires as to whether or not you two are "trying," don't blush delicately or murmur something unintelligible under your breath. Look him in the eye and proudly tell him, "Yes! I'm so glad you asked! Me and Marvin have been doing the Mattress Mambo on a daily basis in our attempt to conceive Baby Marvina! When our efforts have proved successful, you will be the first to know!" That oughtta fix him.

Of course, if you have indeed been "trying" for almost any length of time with no luck yet, you might have to get a little grittier in your personal PR methods. I know one couple who finally told pushy questioners that the husband was sterile. This is a highly effective way of shutting down unwanted conversation. Of course, people will talk. People always talk, though, but it's your business, after all.

Let's say things are going a wee bit slower than you had hoped. Could someone's equipment be malfunctioning? Well, depending on how long you have actually been working on this project, probably not. Normally fertile couples have a 25 percent chance of getting pregnant each cycle and a cumulative pregnancy rate of 75 to 85 percent over the course of one year. Still, some healthy couples can take even longer to get pregnant. Even if you're now in your seventh, eighth, or ninth month of trying, most doctors don't consider looking into possible fertility issues until a full year has elapsed.

Short of medical intervention (and some doctors recommend an overall reproductive evaluation to rule out tubal blockages or low sperm counts; see "The Big [Guy] Chill" later in this chapter), there are a few things you can do to try to boost your fertility.

The Nifty Nine
Ways to Increase Your Chances of Getting Pregnant

1. Relax

How many stories have we all heard about the couple who finally decides to adopt and then—*bing!*—they're pregnant! Listen to what Sherman Silber, M.D., says: "My best recommendation is not to time intercourse too precisely because it can dramatically increase your stress and, ironically, inhibit ovulation. I recommend you do whatever you can to extract yourself from the hectic, sometimes crazy pace of the modern world and make sure you have time for a quality relationship with your partner. This will do more to relieve stress and allow you to ovulate normally than any other 'natural' remedy."[1]

2. Give Your KY the Kibosh

A little tidbit from our scientist friends that might come in handy right about now: Most "personal lubricants" (you gotta love a good euphemism)

The Big (Guy) Chill

The biggest regret of my journalistic career was interviewing a family member about his infertility. Not that it didn't result in a fascinating and informative story or that he isn't a wonderful person. But I will have to face this relative over the Thanksgiving Day dinner table, year after year, knowing what I know...*whew!* Live and learn, they say, and I sure learned *a lot* that day about male infertility.

Which brings me to this illuminating piece of info: *There is always a 50 percent chance—at least—that the problem is the guy's.* So if you feel like you and yours might be facing fertility issues, I beg you, *get your man tested.* So many couples suffer needlessly because they don't think to explore the possibility that the husband has a low sperm count (or no sperm count, as is sometimes the case). In many cases the situation can be remedied with medical intervention, but you first have to see a doctor to figure out what to do.

While you are busy maturing a single egg at the leisurely pace of about one a month, your mate is almost constantly at work producing millions of microscopic sperm. The problem is (or can be), that sperm production is quite sensitive to temperature. "Things" have to stay at a balmy 94 degrees Fahrenheit—about four degrees cooler than normal body temperature. Here are a few tried and true ways for your guy to keep the family jewels cool, calm, and collected:

- Wear boxers, not briefs.
- Wear loose-fitting pants.
- Stay out of the sauna and hot tub.
- Is biking his hobby? Tell him to take up cross-country skiing instead.
- And on that note: Contact sports like hockey and football are also a bad idea during periods of intentional baby making.

are lethal to sperm and mess with the normal interplay of ejaculated sperm and cervical mucus. Most of the time, the vagina's own acid secretions kill sperm unless it's ovulation time, in which case the sperm is actually protected.

3. Get to Know Your Basal Body Temperature

Here's where your body kind of becomes the site of a science experiment, a fact you probably shouldn't dwell on. Keeping in mind Nifty Nine Number One (relax!), try charting both your body temperature and the consistency of your cervical mucus to plot the exact time you'll ovulate. On the first day of your period, take your temperature with a super-exact basal body thermometer and record the results. When your period is finished, note the consistency of your cervical mucus and jot that down too. When your temperature spikes a little and your mucus is kind of like an egg white, it's show time! A simpler method is to buy one of those nifty ovulation predictor kits, or trying the at-home version. Thus…

4. Embark upon the Great Egg Hunt

Not unlike a chicken, we ladies lay eggs, ideally once a month. The big trick is figuring out when those eggs are a-laying, so you can set up a blind date between your flirty Ms. Ovum and his top-rated Swimmers. An ovulation predictor kit can tell you when you're going to ovulate based on a spike in your luteinizing hormone. Those kits aren't cheap (ranging from $20 to $50 a pop), so consider the much cheaper, but perhaps less accurate, do-it-yourself version: Figure out the first date of your last period. Add fourteen days. Then…

5. Buy a Ticket to the Four-Day Festival of Fun and Fertility

If it's going to happen, it will most likely happen between Day Fourteen and Day Eighteen. At this point an egg will reach maturity in one of your ovaries, which releases it into the abdomen, where it's quickly sucked up

"We Just Keep on Trying and Trying and Trying..."

My husband and I have been trying for more than a year to conceive, and I am just heartbroken every month when I get my period. My best friend and my cousin both got pregnant like that, and it's hard for me to watch them get all excited and prepare for their babies. How can I make this a time of deepening my trust in God instead of getting more and more depressed?

—TRYING IN TUSKEGEE

Dear Trying,

Oh, I can relate to how you're feeling! Perhaps my own story will offer you some hope…

Relaxing on a park bench during a warm and sunny July afternoon, my husband Brian and I began to reminisce about my pregnancy and the long months that preceded it. I am currently six months pregnant, and we are daily amazed by this good gift from our heavenly Father.

Brian and I were married four months when, much to my surprise, my maternal instincts and desires began to emerge. Our premarital discussions regarding children had included my insistence that we wait at least two years before we began the process. Well, by our tenth month of marriage, we both decided to discontinue our birth control and "see what happens." I knew very well that many couples must wait a long period of time to conceive, but deep down I thought that we would soon be celebrating a positive pregnancy test. I began to plan the pregnancy—our announcement to family and friends, an investment in a maternity wardrobe, and a due date the following winter.

I was most premature. The months turned into a year, and the second year began. I convinced myself that our hectic lifestyle in California's Bay Area (which included a two-and-a-half-hour daily commute) was the problem and that, once we moved back to Michigan, my body would

(continued on next page)

become instantly fertile. It didn't happen, and I began to "prep" Brian for the possibility of adoption. Needless to say, my emotions were raw with each twenty-eight-day cycle. I would hold my breath and pray that this would be the month. With each period I would cry out to God and ask, "Why?" During this time, every close married friend of mine became pregnant. The Lord used this time to teach me patience and to remind me that I am not the designer of my own destiny. He is—and always will be.

Upon our return to Michigan, in my fifteenth month of attempts, my ob-gyn agreed to perform three initial tests to determine the cause of my fertility problems. He found that my body was not effectively producing the hormone progesterone, and without it, my body would not be able to maintain a pregnancy even if it achieved one. I began a four-month regimen of hormone therapy. Each time, I was disappointed.

In my twentieth month of attempting to get pregnant, at the recommendation of my most fertile sister-in-law, a mother of five, I made an appointment with a fertility specialist. I joked with Brian as we dressed the morning of the appointment that he'd better present himself well so that the doctor would find us worthy of reproducing. Much prayer preceded that appointment, prayer both for wisdom on the doctor's part and patience on ours. The doctor made no promises, but he was very reassuring and made arrangements for further testing. My appointment had been on a Tuesday, and my period was due that Friday. The first test was scheduled for Friday morning so my progesterone levels could be measured. I returned home that morning with a sense of peace and patience unlike I had felt in months and months. I told my mom that I was ready to work with this doctor for the long haul and that my anxious feelings had measurably subsided.

Thursday morning found me at the doctor's clinic taking a blood test to ensure that I was not pregnant before I began the test the following morning. The sweet nurse mentioned the possibility of a pregnancy, and I reassured her that this test was simply to confirm that I had not yet conceived. I left the clinic, ran errands, and arrived home for an afternoon of household chores when the phone rang. My doctor's nurse was calling with my test results, and as I listened half-heartedly, she announced that the test was positive. Just as I had done earlier that day, I tried to convince this nurse that she must have the wrong test results—I simply couldn't be pregnant. Did she have the right file? Could this be? She was just as surprised as I, and she commented that the doctor had not yet done anything for me. My husband and I spent the entire weekend (and beyond) in a state of wonder and amazement. After 20 months of attempts, the Lord had answered our prayers.

Each and every day of this pregnancy (despite the early months of nausea) has been a day of joy and delight in our Father's goodness to us. We have loved every moment of this process, and we can't wait to welcome this little one into the world and to tell him how the Lord blessed us with him/her. Brian and I are both convinced this path the Lord made for us has drawn us closer to Him and to each other, and we are most thankful.

—MARY JO HAAB, MOTHER OF JOSEPHINE, 6 MONTHS OLD

by the nearest fallopian tube, and voila! Ovulation. The average ripe egg has a life span of twenty-four hours, so MAKE HAY WHILE THE SUN SHINES if you get my meaning. (And if you don't, you need a completely different book!)

6. Rearrange As Needed

Forgive me, but I must be quite frank and discuss the very best arrangement of limbs and whatnot for you and your mate during this crucial process. No one knows for sure, but some experts believe the missionary position (man on top) or the rear-entry position (man behind woman, both facing the same direction) are best because they supposedly provide your guy's Swimmers with optimum infiltration. That out of the way, I'd urge you to do whatever you like anyway. The key is to have a good time and to have a good time often enough that live sperm are ready to go into your reproductive track to meet up with Her Excellency the Egg. That means you should...

7. Make Love Every Other Day

Why not every blessed free minute, you might ask. The thing is, when you're trying too hard, your body knows it and will rebel. (I'm starting to feel like Dr. Ruth.) Plus, too much pressure will work against enjoyment. No one wants to be told to drop his trousers at 8:57 P.M., while loading the dishwasher or paying the bills or attending a nephew's tuba recital—or else! I mean, what fun is that? (Although, if you do interrupt the recital, the look on Aunt Mildred's face might have some fun value. The arrest, not so much.)

8. Stare at the Ceiling

Though far from being a scientific fact, some experts say that a woman should stay on her back (with a pillow underneath her south end) for at least twenty to thirty minutes so gravity can help the sperm rendezvous with the egg.

Fabulous Folic Acid

You've got to be extra vigilant about getting certain nutrients for your baby, even now, before he or she has been officially started. Folic acid is one such nutrient that has been getting a lot of attention the last several years, and for good reason. "Folic acid has been shown in many reputable studies to decrease the incidence of birth defects such as spina bifida," says Dr. Mary Beth Grey, D.O., an ob-gyn in private practice in Grand Rapids, Michigan.

The trick with this fabulous nutrient is to get enough of it during the first four weeks of pregnancy when your baby's nervous system is developing. Since many women don't even know they are pregnant until their fourth week, Grey advises taking a multivitamin with folic acid if you are trying to conceive. So start taking a prenatal vitamin with 800 mcg of folic acid (some have only 400 to 600 mcg) as soon as you decide to try for a pregnancy. Also, load up on folate-rich foods until at least the third or fourth month of your pregnancy.

The good news:
- 1/2 cup cereal (fortified): 146-179 mcg
- 4 spears steamed or boiled asparagus: 88 mcg
- Medium-sized papaya: 115 mcg
- 1/2 cup steamed broccoli: 52 mcg
- 1 cup cantaloupe: 27.2 mcg
- Large hard-boiled egg: 22 mcg

The bad news:
- 1/2 cup chicken liver: 539 mcg
- 1/2 cup beef liver: 184.5 mcg
- 1/2 cup lentils: 179 mcg
- 1 oz. wheat germ: 100 mcg

Orange juice has lots of the good stuff, and so does a nice green salad. So, really, no need to gulp down Chicken Liver Lentil Surprise. Unless of course that's your thing.

9. Last But Not Least, Pray

This is an absolutely vital component to trying to get pregnant. This is not to say if you pray God will give you a baby. It may not be in His plan for you to bear biological children. He may have something else in store for you. But even the most secular sources advise women trying to conceive to pray to someone, the reasoning being that those who pray have more calm and less stress. I say, stick with the one true God, the source of unnatural peace and uncanny wisdom. When you focus on His power and goodness, not to mention His constant presence, you will calm down—way down. Abiding close to your Father in heaven will help you stay on His course for your life and attuned to His wisdom. And there's simply no better preparation for parenthood than that.

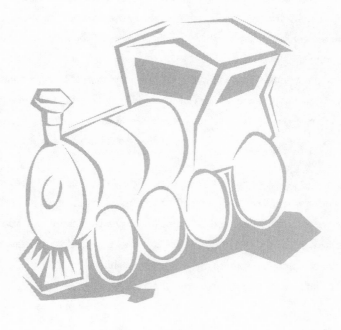

Dear Baby!

I knew it! I just knew it! You are here, despite several negative pregnancy tests. We just got back from Costa Rica, your old dad and me, and I even took a couple of tests along on vacation to see if you had come. I had a funny feeling they were wrong because I kept having to get up in the night and go to the bathroom. And I was soooo emotional about this Elian Gonzalez thing. The television coverage of him being seized by the government was almost traumatic for me, and I really overreacted. Anyway, this is just amazing news, that our little family of three is going to be four (plus of course, Pierre, our cat).

I know you are just itty bitty, and lots of people wouldn't even consider you human yet, but you are my very own baby. I keep thinking that maybe Grandma Loewen knew about you before I did, she being up there in heaven with Jesus. And Aunt Gladys and Lori, my best childhood friend, too. That just blows my mind.

Well, you're probably going to be asking for a tattoo someday, although hopefully not for a while. Here's a deal for you: You can get one, but only if it says, "Made in Costa Rica," and it has to go on the bottom of your foot, okay? (Between you and me, I myself would not be opposed to a small, discreetly placed Canadian flag on my own person. Shhhh.)

I just can't wait to meet you, precious little one.

All my love,
Mama

The Stick, the Stunning, and the Start of a Stupendous Adventure

Dear Father, Our Creator,
You know exactly how our baby's cells are multiplying. You are not only the giver of life; You are also the designer. We commit every intricate detail of our baby's body to You. Strengthen that tiny, tiny heart, which has started to beat. Mold every organ. We thank You for Your tender care....
Amen.

—JOYCE PENNER, *What to Pray When You're Expecting*[1]

Snapshot! You never thought you'd be the mother of a tadpole, but here you are, carrying a vaguely amphibian-looking little lima bean inside of you. Your precious embryo has tiny limb buds, which will grow into arms and legs. (Awwww!) On the twenty-fifth day of your pregnancy, his or her heart starts to beat. (If for some reason you get an early ultrasound, you'll be able to see Baby's heart flickering away like mad.) Pop those prenatals because the all-important neural tube—your baby's future brain and spinal cord—is growing. At the end of the first month, the embryo is about half an inch long and weighs less than an ounce.

Positively Pregnant

You've all seen the commercials on television for home pregnancy tests, the ones where "real" folks anxiously await the results: Will it be a line? Two lines? A geometric shape of some kind? And then, at this incredibly personal moment, the television couple holds the stick up to the camera and reveals that they have become parents. Joy ensues, a tear or two are shed, and the brand spanking new mama and papa embrace. If you find yourself crying along at home, you may have your first clue that *you* are preggers too. Or you may just be premenstrual, which is why they invented home pregnancy tests.

One benefit you'll gain by reading this book is you get to learn from my mistakes. Okay, perhaps these are too numerous to mention, but for your sake I will try to cram them between the covers. Here is the first of my many silly yet well-meaning flub-ups from which you may learn: Even through my second pregnancy (yup, the *second* one), I believed I could find out the very day after "implementation" (another thing you will find out about me is I like to use euphemisms for sex because my parents are likely to read this) whether the sperm and the egg had successfully merged.

This unfounded theory meant that I rang up a hefty bill at the drugstore over the next month. When my husband suggested I wait a little bit ("like a week") so as not to cut into our food budget so much, I just gave him The Look, the withering one that says, "I don't think so" in a hundred different languages. I will grant him that these tests are not cheap. And even though I am sure the generic brands measure Human Chorionic Gonadotropin (the hormone present in your urine that says "oh boy!"— or girl) just as well as the spendier brands (that is, by the guys who pay for the three-hankie television ads), I generally feel compelled to go with the $20 boxes. So if you haven't taken the test yet, take my hard-earned wisdom on the matter: Wait "like a week" plus a couple of days after you ovulate, which should place you about the first day you miss your period. The suspense won't kill you, exactly, and this way you won't have dumped $50 or more into negative tests.

Once you have waited until that moment when your period should be with you and yet is not, choose your test with care. First, read the directions carefully because the instructions vary with the brand. Some require you to urinate in a cup and then, using a dropper, place a small sample into a testing well. Others let you "void" (my nurse mother's favorite technical term) directly onto a stick. Go with the easiest possible route to results— in my opinion, the one-step pee-on-a-stick routine. At a time when your brain may already be somewhat pickled with pregnancy hormones, not to mention preoccupied beyond belief, you don't want to do too much mixing and measuring. If it's a positive result, yahoo! It's extremely rare that a pregnancy test, done correctly, will show a false positive. (False negatives, however, are slightly more common. If your test comes up negative, but you "feel" deep down in your gut that you're pregnant, take the second test in the box or wait a few more days and retest.)

   Read of the Month

Get the amazing book A Child Is Born by Lennart Nilsson. Week by week, month by month, you can see photos of how your baby is developing inside you. You won't believe how beautiful and developed he or she is right now!

Now there are myriad ways to tell your guy that one of his power swimmers forged an alliance with your egg. Yelling and screaming is one fun, tried-and-true way. Crying and mutely nodding your head up and down is another. Just don't gift-wrap the stick and expect the poor guy to know what it means. (For some reason, this method seems to be a popular way to break the big news to the daddy-to-be.)

One woman's test came up positive the night before she left on a business trip. Her husband happened to be coming home from another trip, and they would just miss each other. Having agreed to leave the car at the airport parking lot for her mate, this newly pregnant woman taped her positive test to the parking voucher and left it in the car for the guy to discover. Of course, the poor man was utterly clueless. He took the voucher, test and all, up to the parking lot attendant, explaining with some confusion that his wife had left it for him this way. The attendant (a woman, fortunately) broke the news to him that he was going to be a father.

Another question to ponder at this time: "Now what do I do with this plastic thing?" My recommendation would be to pitch it. After all, you've just recently urinated on it, and it's not exactly suitable for framing. But some new moms have a strong desire to save this momentous, life-changing piece of plastic and paper. At a scrapbooking wingding, I watched the woman next to me happily paste her EPT test into her baby's memory album. Newly pregnant myself, I came a bit unglued at the thought of saving such a thing. But now they make pregnancy tests that can be preserved in your scrapbook, so you have the luxury to choose: pee and paste or pee and pitch. Either way, your life will never be the same.

The Nifty Nine
Telltale Signs That
You Did the Test Right

1. Chest Changes

If your breasts suddenly enlarge for no apparent reason, you could very well be pregnant. (Jodi, a first-time mom, was amazed at her ever-blossoming bosom. "All of a sudden, I could see my breasts in my peripheral vision," she said. "Before, I could barely see them, period!") Ask Loverboy for a second opinion because he will most likely be able to detect the most miniscule increases in your breast size. While he's completing this assignment (one he will take very seriously), you may want to say, "Look but don't touch." Your breasts may be swollen, tender, and oddly heavy: Ouch! Also odd: Your chest may suddenly sprout such a profusion of blue-veined roads and rivers that it will look as if elves from Rand McNally have been visiting you in the night.

2. Bathroom Breaks
According to some sources, we pregnant ones are only supposed to start going to the bathroom more frequently at about six to eight weeks, but I started making more trips even before I knew I was pregnant.

3. General Emotional Instability
Like PMS, pregnancy hormones make you slightly loony and apt to get teary-eyed over things that normally wouldn't be very moving (such as allergy medicine commercials). Also, if you want to rip your husband's head off because he forgot to update the checkbook (never mind the fourteen receipts in your purse), you may not be a complete jerk, just a nice girl with spiked levels of progesterone.

4. Naps
Yawn. All of a sudden, you may feel the irresistible urge to curl up in a ball and have one of those really satisfying, drool-all-over-your-pillow, dead-to-the-world daytime sleeps. If you wake up feeling slightly comatose, drag yourself out of bed to make a sandwich, then really think you should take another nap, you are probably pregnant. If the cat is looking at you condescendingly (of course, when is he not?) as if to say, "You sluggish slob," you know things are not normal.

5. Extra Spit
This is one of the first, but definitely not the last, in a series of bizarre, freakish, albeit normal symptoms: Many pregnant women produce massive amounts of saliva. Lest you think you are in the beginning stages of rabies, take heart.

6. Fainting and Prefainting Spells

I have never personally fainted, although it has always held a certain dramatic allure. Pregnant pals, though, have reported that the world can sometimes spin in the most dizzying fashion even before their pregnancy test comes up positive.

7. Pained Innards

For me, in the days just before I find out I am indeed with child, I feel as if I have a really wicked case of PMS, including that crampy, oh-boy-here-we-go-again feeling. It's like cramps unplugged: You feel 'em, for sure, but you know the real thing packs a way higher voltage. In this case, though, the pain will take about nine more months to really live up to—and exceed—its promise.

8. Queasiness

Something is rotten in Denmark—or at least it sure smells that way to you. Suddenly just the teensiest waft of food odors from down the hall may hit you like a Mack truck and send you careening toward the nearest toilet. (Of course, if you took your vitamins on an empty stomach this morning, that could cause nausea too.)

9. No period

Well, duh. If you are one of those women who gets her period so regular-like that you can set your watch to it, the absence of said symptom should be considered pretty suspicious, especially when added to the other eight signals. Congratulations, new mama!

Feelings, Whoa, Whoa, Whoa...

Upon finding out that you are indeed pregnant, you'll also find that you have to deal with a huge jumble of emotions. Few other moments in life hold the drama, the portentousness, the hurricane of intense feelings, all swirling together in a dizzying storm, that this moment does. Hopefully, you're sitting down for much of this maelstrom of emotion. Maybe you could light a candle (one of those overpriced things you bought at your sister-in-law's candle party) and take some time to begin to think and pray about the overwhelming wonder of being pregnant. My motto is, aromatherapy can't hurt. Don't worry if the pink candle promises to "soothe and relax" and the green one is supposed to "rejuvenate and restore." Just light something and have a seat.

 ## Cyber Bulletins

As soon as a physician confirms your pregnancy, sign up at BabyCenter.com for weekly email updates on your pregnancy and your baby's development. You'll look forward to these nifty cyber bulletins, which keep you up-to-date with breaking news for both of you. (Similar services are provided by ThatGlow.com and FitPregnancy.com.)

You're in shock, girl.

The stunned feeling is a definite, whether you and your guy have been trying to conceive for what seems like eons or this is a complete and utter failure of your fail-safe birth-control method. (For the latter group, skip the candles and go directly to the smelling salts, which, by the way, should not be lighted.) The fact that you are really, truly pregnant is quite simply unbelievable. Assuming you are totally freaked, you may be feeling any number of things.

If you planned your pregnancy, even longed for it, you are probably profoundly happy, elated that this dream of yours and your husband's has come true. You know God has given you this incomparable, sweet, and lavish gift. The verse "Every good and perfect gift is from above, coming down from the Father of the heavenly lights" (James 1:17) keeps running through your mind. Like a broken record, you keep saying—out loud or in your mind—"Thank You, thank You, thank You!" He hears you, and I know He's smiling. You are His daughter, and He loves to give you joy.

But rarely is joy isolated from other emotions. (We mortals are just way too complicated.) There is also fear—and fear's insidious offspring, worry. I recently met a woman in her early twenties, Blythe, in the baby-name section of a bookstore. Figuring she was pregnant (what else would she be doing there?), I struck up a conversation. She had just found out she was expecting. Just. In fact, she hadn't even been to the doctor's for the confirming blood test. "I'm really excited," she told me. "But I'm also really scared something will go wrong with the baby." You could see the warring emotions all over her cute face.

The fear is there, I think, because right off the bat the stakes are high. After all, it's your baby, your son or daughter, inside of you. And you have been immediately seized with such profound love, such a delicious, heady feeling of adoration. Blythe's baby was, at that moment, no bigger than a grain of rice, teeny, shapeless, and looking more like a baby frog than a baby human. But love was exuding out of this new mommy's every pore, even the pores plugged up with her nose ring. She loved this child she was carrying, and love carries with it the risk of loss.

You know how much you feel for your baby already. If something were to happen, the loss would hurt. Fifteen to 20 percent of pregnancies do end in miscarriage. But don't let the fear of what might happen dampen the joy and the love and the fabulousness of these early weeks. And don't hold back your love in an effort to protect your own heart. Even if the very worst should happen and you do lose your baby, you will know that you loved that child with all your heart. The reward of that experience should last for all time. And imagine that grand and beautiful day in heaven when you hold your child in your arms.

During both of my pregnancies, I prayed a prayer something like this: "Lord, You know I am so delirious with happiness I could pop. But You also know better than anyone that I am already afraid of losing this precious baby. Help me to understand in a deeper way that You are in charge

"What If He's Not So Excited About This?"

I'm not entirely sure my husband is going to be happy about the news I am pregnant. I myself am thrilled, but I am worried about his reaction. How can I break the news to him with tact, and how can I avoid feeling resentment toward him if he is not as excited as I am?

—WORRIED IN WYOMING

Dear Worried,

When Troy and I married, we planned our future out to the smallest detail. We were going to study, work hard, and finish school. Then, with degrees in hand, we would work in our related fields. Gradually, we would invest in a home and a second car. Once all our ducks were in a row, we would think about having children.

We wanted children, just not right away. We needed time—lots of time, mind you—to grow in our marriage and get "established" before we could take on the added responsibility of raising a family. But God had other ideas. He wanted us to trust in Him with all our lives, hopes, and plans. In the process of learning to trust in God, we also had to learn to trust in each other.

But trusting each other to be tender and gracious when our plan backfired was another story. I didn't think Troy could handle changes, especially one this big, in our sacred plans. When I began to suspect that I was pregnant, I realized how little I trusted Troy—and God.

My sister and I had this silly little tradition: Whenever my period was late, I would call her. Then I would call her back when it came. It was a goofy way for two sisters to keep some semblance of contact across the miles. This time, however, was different. I waited longer than usual to call Esther, feeling deep down that I was indeed pregnant. Then, each day for almost two weeks, I called and said my period had still not arrived. She urged me to tell Troy, but I was scared.

(continued on next page)

Finally, it was crunch time. I had tried to drop hints and work my way into the topic, but that only made things worse. One night, just before he drifted off to sleep, I asked him, "Troy, what would be the top three things you would fear the most right now?"

"If you were to die." (Well, yeah, pretty understandable.)

"If we were to get a divorce." (Two down, but number three was what I was dreading.)

"If you were pregnant."

"Oh," I managed and quietly cried myself to sleep.

The next day I knew I had to tell him. When he came home from work, I sat him down on the couch and launched into the speech I had been preparing all day. (Did I mention this was also exam week?) Before I was even halfway done, Troy blurted out his suspicion. "You're pregnant, aren't you?" When I burst into tears, he took me in his arms and told me that everything was going to be okay.

All that time I had spent withholding my trust from him, worrying and building up my courage had only led to feelings of inadequacy, fear, and rejection. But when I opened myself up to Troy, he had an excellent opportunity to show me his love and his trustworthiness. I don't know how your husband will react, but I do know it's better to trust him with the news rather than get all worked up.

In some ways our second pregnancy was an even greater blow to our "plan." We had barely gotten a handle on our new life with our firstborn, Jonathan, a young toddler, when we sat in a doctor's office and heard the shocking news that my pregnancy test was positive. Troy interrupted the doctor's well-worn oration on prenatal vitamins, nutrition, and so on.

"So when you say the test is positive, does that mean she is positively not pregnant or positively pregnant?"

"Oh, she's positively pregnant," the doctor clarified.

"But she can't be pregnant! We just got everything under control! I'm in a master's program, and she's going to be a teacher soon. Everything is finally going according to plan!"

After the doctor picked up his jaw off the floor, he wrote me a prescription for prenatals and sent us on our way. Again, we were reminded of our need to fully trust God. Once we settled in to trust mode again, our joy soon followed. In trusting God, we can find joy in His promises. Obediently living out His joy and aspirations for us is what makes our lives truly fulfilling.

By the time we were expecting our third surprise from the Lord, we had our trust issues under control. We are now blessed with three wonderful boys. I have never used my teaching degree in a classroom, but I am beginning to homeschool our six-year-old son. Troy worked many long hours trying to support his family and finish his master's degree at night. Our lives have never really wound back to our original plan, but we decided we like what God has done even better.

Pregnancy is a trusting process, and trusting is a pregnant process, full of morning sickness, groaning, stretching, backaches, surprises, hope, joy, and love. Love enough to trust—and trust enough to give of yourself. These are the blessings that come only from the Lord! He will fulfill His promise to "make your paths straight" (Proverbs 3:6).

—JULIANNA CLINK, MOTHER OF JONATHAN, 7,
NATHANIEL, 5, AND DARNELL, 3

here. Nothing is going to happen to my baby or me unless it is in Your plan for us. If something is going to happen—and You know everything—I pray that You will prepare my heart for whatever it is. Help me to relax in knowing that Your grace is enough to cover any hurt, and help me to enjoy this treasure with every ounce of my being."

Make it a habit, day by day, hour by hour, to give your worries to God. And then give yourself up to the pure exultation. Grab your guy and celebrate in some goofy, joyful way. Go to the nearest bookstore-café, order a decaf mocha latté, and browse the baby-name section. Hit the mall and ooh and ahh over snuggly little baby outfits. Tell the dog he's going to be a "big brother" and then cry because that cute, droopy-eared fleabag isn't going to be your baby anymore. (Don't deny it. Ever since Fido came into your house as a puppy, you've been pouring all your maternal energies into him.)

If your husband gives you a funny look, hug him and tell him to get used to random fits of weeping. Then place your first takeout and delivery order. You're pregnant, for Pete's sake, and all of a sudden, you have the worst craving for a Butterfinger Blizzard.

What to Do This Month

☐ If you haven't selected a physician to help see you through your pregnancy, get a recommendation from a trusted friend. No one can give you a better referral than a friend who has a positive partnership with her doc. Physician referral services can also help you find a doctor who works in your area and is accepted by your insurance carrier.

☐ Make your first appointment, which will usually take place around your tenth week.

☐ Ask your physician or OB to prescribe a prenatal vitamin for you.

☐ Think about whom you want to tell and how soon. Some people opt to wait until they are twelve weeks along in case of a miscarriage. I myself could hardly wait more than a few hours, but that's just me.

☐ Be mindful of things you eat and drink (more on this in chapter 3). Cut down on caffeine, and stay away from alcohol completely. It's not just about you anymore!

☐ Begin a journal to your baby. Start by sharing how thrilled you are to find out you are carrying him. Be sure to describe how his daddy received the good news.

Dear Baby,

I'm trying, I really am, sweetness. But it's really hard to take those huge and potent prenatals the way my stomach has been lately. At least I know I am definitely pregnant, what with throwing up four times a day! Well, this is starting to sound like a guilt trip, and it's definitely not. (I'll save that for when you're a teenager, and then the whole morning-sickness story will sound like something out of science fiction.) I am so happy you are with me, even though it means making the bathroom my new headquarters.

Oma and Opa are so excited too, but they are really hoping you'll have a cousin soon. I think they are worried about Uncle Dan and Aunt Tina, although I think those two will surprise us with an announcement any day now. We invited Grandma and Grandpa Craker over, and I made them this card with a picture of your big brother Jonah (we all call him Jo Jo) "reading" the newspaper. On the front it said, "Read all about it," and then inside, "I'm going to have a baby brother or sister under my Christmas tree." I pasted a magazine picture of a newborn in there, and I placed a hockey-stick sticker in its hand. Oh, and the baby had skates on too. Hope you like hockey! Grandma and Grandpa were surprised—and happy, too.

Anyway, baby doll, as we spread the word, we are getting more and more psyched. So you hang in there with me, and I will do my utmost to keep down my vitamins. For now, I gotta take a nap!

Love,
Mama

Nausea, Narcolepsy, and General Nuttiness

I would cry at AT&T commercials. I'd be sobbing and Johnny would say, "What's wrong?" and I'd say "The g-g-g-grandfather got to see his g-g-g-grandson!"

—KELLY PRESTON, actress and wife of John Travolta, talking about hormonal fluctuations during pregnancy

Snapshot! You and baby are officially connected! The placenta and the umbilical chord are fully operative by week five, passing nutrients and oxygen between you and Junior. Baby has grown to one inch long and has distinct, slightly webbed fingers, and his veins are clearly visible. His heart, about the size of a poppy seed, is divided into right and left chambers, and it is beating away. At eight weeks, your one-ounce wonder now boasts a brain, spinal cord, and a teeny little baby bum. Baby's squirming too—but you can't feel it yet!

It's Not Easy Being Green

I will never forget my first bout with morning sickness. I happened to be traveling in Europe, fulfilling a lifelong dream before I would fulfill another longtime wish: to become a mother. I was about seven weeks pregnant, and between jet lag and first-trimester fatigue, I felt anything but perky. I was visiting my friend Susan in Madrid, where she was teaching English. One morning we got up early to tour Spain's royal palace. My stomach felt a bit unsettled, so I skipped breakfast and gulped down a glass of orange juice, settling for a folic acid fix. (I had forgotten my prenatal vitamins—can you believe that? At the time, orange juice was the only sure source of folic acid I could think of, so I drank gallons of it on my trip.)

Bad idea. Take it from me: Never skip breakfast or let your tummy get empty. Force-feed yourself with Saltines if you have to! And, better yet, don't EVER drink orange juice on an empty stomach!

So there we were, Sue and I, trying gamely to decipher the tour guide's broken English as we walked from one opulent chamber to the next, every wall echoing with the voices of past kings and queens. Just as I was able to make out the words "priceless carpets," I felt a sensation so alarming, so potentially catastrophic, that all I could do was grip the velvet rope partition with white knuckles. I was definitely going to spew my insides all over King Juan Carlos's throne room. Visions of irritated royal carpet tenders flashed through my head, as did the irrational yet piercing thought, *What if they make me pay for damages?* Well, ice-cold fear shot through my very being—along with the most fervent foxhole prayer I have ever prayed—and the rising nausea miraculously froze in its bilious tracks.

All that to say, you never know when morning sickness is gonna hit. It probably won't be at a convenient time or in a convenient place. I have heard tales of p.g. ladies upchucking in airports, restaurants, malls, at the side of the road, church… One never knows when a blast of HCG will make you feel as if you've just ingested seven lemons on an empty stomach.

Here's a story that made me cringe for the poor woman: A Kmart cashier was violently nauseated one day on her shift, so much so that she couldn't make a quick enough exit when her stomach started its shake, rattle, and roll. So there she was, trapped behind the counter. To add insult to injury, a pushy customer was berating her for some retailing issue that wasn't even remotely her fault. This poor pregnant woman did the only thing she could: She knelt down right where she was and heaved into a

Kmart bag. Not only did her customer not immediately melt with compassion, but the woman continued to complain loudly without even missing a beat. Think of this story next time you're hurling your guts in the privacy of your own bathroom—and count your blessings.

Writer Susan Maushart, in her book *The Mask of Motherhood*, compares her expectations of morning sickness to the stunning reality of her own experience: "I expected 'mild nausea' that 'vomiting would instantly relieve.' What I got was a sickness so intense that it disordered my senses. I would not have believed (had I not experienced it) that music, for example, could be experienced as an acute physical irritation. There are still some rhapsodies of Rachmaninoff that affect me like the aftertaste of tainted seafood. At the time, even my ears wanted to throw up."[1]

Despite my near-miss experience in the royal palace, my first pregnancy wasn't too bad when it came to morning sickness. I mean, I thought it was bad, but little did I know how bad it could really get. With my second baby, I was really, truly, riotously trapped in a vortex of almost nonstop nausea. According to mothering myth, if you find yourself spending undue amounts of time with your face in the toilet, you are

Ann B's Handy-Dandy Roadside Emergency Kit

My friend Ann is currently pregnant with her first child. As she passed through the morning-sickness phase, she came up with this great, super-practical idea for handling those oh-so-inconvenient close encounters of the queasy kind. "In the car, I packed a little plastic bucket with really sturdy zip-lock bags, tissues, wet wipes, bottled water, and mouthwash. That way when I felt like throwing up, I could just pull over, do the deed, throw the bag out, drink some water, and swish with mouthwash. Thankfully, I've only needed it once—so far!"

going to have a girl. Some of my friends swear this is true; others say they were just as queasy or sicker yet when they were pregnant with a boy.

My own two-year-old boy thought it was great fun when I began to make my regular dash upstairs to unfurl my insides. Here I thought the poor little tyke would be scared by the dramatic noises, but in a spirit of *joie de vivre* he joined the game in his own way. He would race up the stairs after me and stand like a little soldier behind me, patting my back. "You gotta puke, Mommy?" he would say as I heaved. As soon as I was finished and splashing water on my face, the whole thing would strike him as hilarious, and he would begin to imitate me, emitting the most unearthly, guttural vomiting noises I've ever heard. He even parlayed this skill into a party trick, regaling friends, family, and, once, patrons of a Chinese restaurant—who began to look dimly at their Dim Sum—with the loud announcement, "Mommy puked!" followed by an encore performance of retching noises. At least one of us was having a good time.

Morning sickness and its resulting upheaval of breakfast, lunch, and dinner lead to one of the great paradoxes of pregnancy. Pregnancy Paradox One: How are you supposed to provide a colorful array of nutrients for Baby when you can't even keep down a piece of unbuttered toast? Many women worry that by vomiting they are depriving their fetus of essential vitamins. Mary Beth Grey, my very own ob-gyn and the mother of two little boys, offers this (somewhat) reassuring news: "As long as you can eat during the day at some point, you will probably do okay. The baby will suck what it needs from you—you will be the one to suffer if you don't eat properly. The baby will still get what it needs unless you have a real prolonged period where you can't keep anything down at all."

Ruth de Boer-Logi, a clinical dietician at Spectrum Health in Grand Rapids, Michigan, suggests to pregnant women who suffer from morning sickness that they eat small, frequent meals in order to keep something in their stomachs. "At the hospital, we have a diet for women who have hyperemesis, which means they are throwing up constantly," she says. "We give them some kind of dry food, and then an hour later some liquids, and then another hour later a solid-food snack of some kind," and so on. In extreme cases, women with hyperemesis have to be hospitalized and monitored due to dehydration and weight loss. But Ruth and Dr. Grey agree that extreme cases of hyperemesis are rare.

Especially if you are a first-time mom, the anxiety caused by the nutrition for the baby issue alone is enough to make you queasy. On the one hand, it has been strongly suggested that you discard all junk food and nosh all the livelong day on lentils and hydroponic spinach. On the other hand, you may sense that the only foods having a remote chance of passing the vomit barrier are Count Chocula cereal and Velveeta sandwiches. Fortunately, all is not lost. I am a firm believer in trying your best and letting that be good enough. (More on big-picture nutrition in the next chapter.) If you follow a few time-honored "mommalies" for coping with morning sickness, you and the baby should be just fine:

    ## Think Bland, Very Bland

No, not for the baby's name or the nursery décor, but for the foods you attempt to stomach during the peak morning-sickness period, weeks 7 to 14. Try Saltines, breadsticks, yogurt, and pretzels, and forgo spicy and fatty foods—for now, anyway. Around month four you will return, with a vengeance, to the habit of eating. And *how!*

First, eat crackers first thing in the morning. Keep simple snacks, such as Goldfish crackers, by your bedside. When you wake up, nibble a few crackers and then, if possible, rest for twenty to thirty minutes before getting out of bed. Of course, if you actually have a job to get to or one or two hungry mouths to feed (not including your husband, who should be making his own breakfast by now), skip the twenty minutes of morning relaxation and munch the crackers.

Second, don't swallow your prenatal vitamin on an empty stomach or, preferably, in the morning at all. Popping those huge, potent vitamins (my cowboy father-in-law says they look like horse pills) first thing in the morning with nothing bland and yeasty to buffer the acids is a recipe for disaster. You will be visiting the loo *toute de suite!* Try to save your vitamin for just before you go to bed. Then take it with a cup of milk and some crackers or toast. I had the most non-nausea success with this method.

Third, eat what sounds good. I've heard many pregnant women confess that the only thing that sounds good can be obtained via a drive-through window and accompanied by the phrase, "Would you like fries with that?" For me, a Quarter Pounder with cheese was about the only thing that could tame my queasiness. It made me feel better, which then made me more able to eat more nutritious foods that also sounded palatable, like cottage cheese and strawberries. Of course, I ended up gaining weight despite the fact that I threw up four times a day for two months straight, but at least I was able to eat a few good-for-me foods and—this is key— take my prenatal once a day and keep it down.

Nap Attacks

Pregnancy Paradox Two (of several hundred): How am I supposed to stay awake fourteen or fifteen hours a day when I can't even have a cup of coffee in the morning?! Well, actually you can have one cup, but I'll get to that later in the next chapter. The point here is, in your first trimester, you will experience the most mind-numbing, pervasive, and overpowering fatigue of your entire life. One of the most fascinating aspects of cat ownership is to watch the kitty suddenly nod off at all hours of the day and night, as if tranquilized. Forgive an apparent non sequitur: One minute the critter is climbing the drapes, and the next he's stone cold *out*. According to my husband, a Bill Nye the Science Guy wannabe, felines do have some sort of chemical in their brain which dopes them up regularly. As for you, you have an even better excuse than Frisky: You're growing a human being!

In *What to Expect When You're Expecting,* the authors write: "In some ways, your pregnant body is working harder even when you're resting than a non-pregnant body is when mountain climbing. For one thing, your body is manufacturing your baby's life support system."[2] That life support system is your placenta, which will be under construction until about your fourth month. Plus, your hormone levels and metabolism are rapidly changing while your blood sugar and blood pressure tend to be lower. All of this contributes to your fatigue.

 A Good Reason for Morning Sickness?

According to a British medical study reported in the May 2000 issue of *Obstetrics and Gynecology,* there may actually be a good medical reason for morning sickness. Researchers discovered that insulin production increases during the first part of pregnancy. Insulin regulates Mom's blood sugar and is usually released by her body in response to the food that she eats. When insulin levels and levels of insulin growth factor-1 (IGF-1) are spiked in the mother's bloodstream, she metabolizes more fat—at the expense of the developing baby, say the researchers. Thus, morning sickness is thought to keep the amount of food in the mother's bloodstream to a minimum, thereby keeping insulin levels low and slowing the increased metabolism of fat. This helps ensure that the fetus gets the nutrients it needs.

According to the study, one of the reasons that morning sickness usually goes away after the first trimester is because, as the pregnancy progresses, IGF-1 alone becomes the key to the fetus's growth. Thus, it is no longer necessary for Mom's body to suppress insulin levels. As additional support for their theory, researchers pointed to several studies that indicate women with no morning sickness have higher rates of miscarriage and more underweight babies.

I don't know about you, but the mountain climbing analogy made me feel kind of smug. Sure your old college roommate—she of the rippled abs and taut calves—is, according to her latest postcard, scaling some sort of alp somewhere. But you, clever girl, are manufacturing a full-functioning uber-system, which will pass oxygen and nutrients between you and your child!

You need more sleep.

Well, yeah. But how do you get it? For one thing, some stuff will just have to go. As previously mentioned, you are currently performing a constant physical workout the likes of which would bring the Detroit Red Wings to their knees (and this is true even if you are watching *The Price Is Right* in your jammies). Everyone—your boss, your husband, your toddler—will just have to understand. Of the three, your toddler will be the least understanding, not knowing what a placenta is or how that could possibly make the slightest difference in his life. Of course, he may also take a nap, which is good news for you.

It's a toss-up between working women and stay-at-home moms as to who gets the short end of the stick during the first-trimester-fatigue period. Working women have to dress themselves, shower, and eat breakfast—enough activity to induce a nap right there. But then they have to produce lucid ideas and linear trains of thought for the next eight hours. When I was working, I used to find my pregnant pal Lisa passed out on her desk, utterly sedated. If you have an office with a door, you could possibly indulge in a couple of fifteen- to twenty-minute power naps. Now that she has two little ones at home and is pregnant for the third time, Lisa swears it is easier to snatch a snooze than it was when she was working. She waits for her two-year-old to take his nap, pops in a movie for her four-year-old, and sleeps for a good hour a day.

If you work and don't already have other kids at home, clear your evening schedule and plan on turning in soon after supper. John, a newspaper editor, tells of how his then-pregnant wife, Pam, used to come home after a long day working in a daycare center: "'I'm too tired for dinner,' she would say. I'd reply, 'Oh, don't worry about that, honey. I can make dinner.' Then she'd say, 'No, you don't understand. I'm too tired to eat.'"

If you are at home with one, two, or more munchkins running around, good luck. My friend Amy recently experienced her fourth pregnancy—and three little ones under the age of five at home! "I just got them on a schedule of napping, or at least quiet time," she says. "Even the oldest would be quiet for an hour or so, and I just slept because I absolutely had to." If you are the type that can nap in front of a television (my husband, for example, cannot have a siesta unless there is a football game or the Discovery Channel yammering on the tube), pop in a video and tell your tyke, "Mommy is tired, and I need you to watch your movie quietly." Obviously, this works better with a child closer to age three than with a one-year-old. But this is a time in your life when you need to beg, borrow, and steal snatches of sleep.

Snooze Time

These nap attacks are real, biological, bona fide ways for your body to get the rest it needs. This is no time to be tough! You—and Baby—need the extra ZZZs.

If your parents live nearby and are willing and able to help, call them for emergency babysitting. Hire the thirteen-year-old in your neighborhood to come over every afternoon for an hour or two and watch your older child while you sleep. Your husband may be your greatest resource. Impress upon him your urgent need to get extra sleep (toss the word *placenta* around freely) and have him cover some dinners and weekend childcare duties if he's not doing so already.

Some women report going from one extreme to another, from severe narcolepsy to bouncing off the ceilings. "You may wake one morning with enough energy to rearrange your cabinets, iron your husband's underwear, and slice blades of grass to give your lawn a more lush appearance," says writer Karen Vogel. "Then, you'll drop exhausted on the couch, swearing off even the most mundane tasks for the rest of the day, only to be recharged in an hour and ready to spit shine your bathroom floor."[3]

I myself never experienced any such fluctuations in energy. I was on one speed and one speed only for three months: precomatose. But, like most aspects of pregnancy, the good news is that this, too, shall pass. When that droopy, draggy feeling passes during your second trimester, you will wonder if you were in fact babying yourself during months one through three or four. Could you have really been that sleepy? But then, in the beauty of God's design, just so you don't overdo it in the homestretch, the drugged feeling will make an encore appearance in your seventh month. At that point you can reread this chapter—or just take another nap. Look to the cat for moral support. Even if no one else does, he understands.

C'mon, Get Sappy:
The Emotional Tilt-a-Whirl, Part 1

Know this my pregnant friend: Your hormone levels won't change gradually. Instead, upon conception, you will be struck by a progesterone thunderbolt. Not unlike being struck by lightning, you will crackle and buzz and generally convulse uncontrollably as this force of nature riddles your body. It may sound dramatic, but trust me: Until you've wept at the Ice Capades as I have, you don't know PMS from PHS (Pregnancy Hormonal Syndrome).

There I was, taking notes on the production for my newspaper review, thinking this was a pleasant, amusing, and engaging family event (though the skating itself was nothing the Lithuanian Olympic judge would give a fig for). Then the finale began, and all the characters from previous numbers gathered on the ice for a rousing close. Suddenly it struck me that these characters, including Ariel from The Little Mermaid, Jasmine from Aladdin, and (oddly enough) representatives from some science-fiction film, were like a microcosm of the people of the world, now working together in a spirit of goodwill and bonhomie. Could world peace, I wondered, be far off if such a disparate group could join hands and occasionally perform double axels simultaneously? Tears streamed down my face as my companion looked at me with some alarm. Moments later, when the storm passed, I wondered if I had finally flipped my lid.

Writer Karen Vogel recalls feeling a tad nutty during her pregnancy. "I cried at Hallmark commercials. I cried at diaper commercials. I cried when I spoke with my mother on the telephone," she writes. "For heaven's sake, I cried ripping an envelope one day because it symbolized the death of a tree."[4]

Sarah and her husband were at a weekend retreat with a bunch of young couples from their church when she experienced the emotional tilt-a-whirl: "We were all playing Taboo, and it was just a really fun, casual atmosphere. But I just felt so out of it. I wasn't getting anything in this game. My husband underestimated how sensitive I was, and he started laughing at me and teasing me—totally in good nature. But I just burst into tears. Everyone just stared at me as I was having this total breakdown over nothing. No one knew how to react. Then all of the sudden, it struck me as hilarious, and I started laughing as hard as I had been crying. Pretty soon everyone was laughing with me."

One more reality check for you. My friend Ellen is normally a stable, calm, and composed woman who doesn't let her emotions get the better of her. Now that she is in her second pregnancy, though, she is experiencing some odd mood swings. "In the last few months I have been more anxious and paranoid about things than I ever have in my whole life. I feel so big and unattractive—asexual almost—and I wonder how my husband could possibly be attracted to me anymore. I even think really irrational thoughts, like, *Now I am going to have two kids. What if my marriage falls apart and I have to support them, with me being a stay-at-home mom?*

When hormones don't besiege her, Ellen knows full well that her marriage is strong and her body isn't a turn-off to her husband. "But it's awful to feel this paranoia," she says.

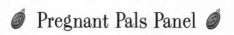

"What Should I Tell My Coworkers?"

I work in a high-pressure office situation, and I'm not sure how or when to tell my coworkers about my pregnancy. Although I am excited to be pregnant, I just don't know what to think about my job. Will my coworkers and boss look at me differently, or maybe even pass me over for a promotion because of it?

—CORPORATELY CONFUSED IN CLEVELAND

Dear Confused,

I remember wondering how the news of my pregnancy—an unexpected one—would be received and whether my career would suffer somehow because of it. I work as a futures trader in Chicago at the Chicago Board of Trade, definitely a high-pressure environment. The first person I told was my boss. At the time she was located in New York and since I wanted a little privacy when telling her, I decided to call her at home. I remember the conversation vividly.

It was a Friday evening in January, and I was quite nervous. I was relatively new on the job, working nights, and I knew it would be difficult to get someone to fill in while I was on maternity leave. I had given the company a commitment to work the off-hours, and I felt I would be letting down my superiors. My boss was a fireball. I knew she had kids of her own, but I did not know her very well. In my opinion she was all about being corporate. She was something of a role model (okay, I idolized her), and I thought my pregnancy would throw everything off track.

Her reaction was as incredible as it was unexpected. She was literally thrilled for me. Gone was Ms. Corporate: I was talking to the mom, the woman. I realized that I was in the best situation, that I had a dream boss. I was so grateful that she was a woman and a mother.

If I had any reservations about the pregnancy affecting my ranking, they flew out the window when she told me how her superior (and thereby mine) had given her a big promotion the very day she told him she was pregnant with her second child. He had been generous and understanding with her about maternity leave, too, so at that moment those kinds of concerns basically became a nonissue for me. She told me to take every day off they gave me and to not worry about anything other than my baby and myself.

This is also the best advice I could give to any pregnant woman in a career. No matter how your boss and coworkers respond, you've got to remember that your baby is the most important thing. Also, if the response is negative and you think your job may be affected, remember that it is discrimination to withhold a promotion or raise from an employee because she is pregnant. Research your rights under the law. Even better, fish around the office for info on how previously pregnant women at the same company have fared.

As I contemplate my next pregnancy, I have to confess being a little paranoid about my news coinciding with year-end bonuses, so I'd like to avoid that if possible. My previous boss is gone, and I now report to a man. News of a pregnancy may or may not go over as well this time around. Also, we're short-staffed, so I imagine filling in for me will be more difficult. (But I know from my first experience that this isn't my concern.)

One issue I may muster up the nerve to address, though, is pumping at work upon my return. Last time I was relegated to the bathroom only to be charged at by a roach on at least one horrifying, breast-milk-went-flying-everywhere occasion. But that's a whole different topic! I really enjoyed my experience of being pregnant, and I can't wait to be pregnant again.

—NANCY RUBIN, 32, MOTHER OF EVA, 3

In general, we human beings are socialized to keep our emotions to ourselves—as much as possible anyway. If someone hurts our feelings at the office, we wait until we're locked in a bathroom stall before sniffling and blowing our noses. If someone cuts us off on the road, we grit our teeth, and though we may rage inwardly, we don't usually scream bloody murder at the culprit. But during pregnancy, the veil between our emotions and our actions, the barrier that separates our inner feelings and the outer self we present to the world, is often pretty thin.

"Lord, Be Her Leaning Post"

Amy Grant once said that every good quality has a dark side, and I think the reverse is also true: Every dark experience has its bright facets. Whether we feel angry at the slightest provocation, irritated and impatient, or prone to crying jags completely disproportionate to the cause (such as television commercials), it's difficult and frustrating to lose control. For some pregnant women, the instability and hormonal wackiness are the most unsettling, even disturbing, aspects of pregnancy.

Read of the Month

Pick up a copy of *What to Pray When You're Expecting* by Joyce Penner. It's a wonderful spiritual companion for this most incredible journey!

But there is one definite bonus to the highly charged emotional state of pregnancy: Never before have we felt so weak, so graceless, and so attacked by our own feelings. And just how is that a bonus, you ask. In such a place of misery, confusion, and instability, there is only one person to whom we can reach out who won't regard us as certifiable: Jesus. He wants us to come to Him with our souls laid bare, with no pretenses or clichés or illusions about our own strength. The beauty of these pregnancy-induced hormonal attacks—and the beauty of the general stress of becoming a new mom, taking on a new role, new responsibilities, and a new life!—is that, in your weakness, God is strong. He wants to comfort you, to put His arms around you, and lift you and carry you through the craziness.

Once not long ago I went up to the front of my church for prayer. A saintly older African American man held my hands in his and prayed a prayer I will never forget. "Lord," he said, not knowing my particular need at that moment, "be her leaning post." It was the perfect thing to say, a beautiful and stalwart image of the stability God offers His children.

No matter how shaky you feel, no matter how swayed and buffeted, you do have a place you can go to, a God who is your refuge and strength. In this unique time of life, what a perfect opportunity to hand the whole mess right over to Him and to hold on to your "leaning post" for dear life.

Praying Through Your Pregnancy

Joyce Penner, author of *What to Pray When You're Expecting*, helps mommies-to-be deepen their faith, trust, and love for God by guiding them through nine months of specific prayer. "Praying for both the physical and spiritual development of our child prepares us emotionally for the transition into parenthood," she writes.[5] Petitioning your heavenly Father not only strengthens your relationship with Him, but working the discipline of prayer into your pregnancy enriches your experience. An added bonus: Because you can't safely assume that your child will follow you in your faith, now is a great time to intentionally nurture her spiritual formation.

Here are some of Joyce's suggestions for specific prayers for yourself as well as your baby during your pregnancy:

- For sensitivity toward childless friends, in both breaking the news and sharing your pregnancy with them.
- For ways to validate your love for your other children, to affirm that they are special to you.

- For good decision making and self-discipline when it comes to getting good nutrition, adequate rest, appropriate exercise—and avoiding those things you know to be harmful to your baby and you.
- For wisdom in protecting, nurturing, and developing the sexuality of your baby right from the start, even before you know whether it's a boy or a girl. Thank God for the gender of the child and ask for acceptance and joy if you hoped for the other gender.
- That the baby may, even in the early stages of gestation, feel you and your husband's love and acceptance.
- For willingness to lay aside your dreams for God's greater purposes.
- For wisdom in tenderly training your child to cherish his or her unique spirit.

The Nifty Nine Ways to Get a Grip

1. Tell Your Guy How You Feel

Tell him in as much detail as you can muster that you feel impatient, overly irritated, suddenly sad—and that you have no idea whatsoever why you were crying. Tell him that you feel out of control and that it would really help if he took your hormonal condition into consideration before reacting to your moods. If your husband knows what to expect, he will be much more at ease even when you are acting like a lunatic.

2. Talk to Your "Yo-Yo Sisters"

No one knows the frustration of coping with torrential emotions like a pal, especially one who has been pregnant or, better yet, is with child this blessed minute. Maybe she will divulge a divine secret of the yo-yo sisterhood, or maybe she will just say, "Poor you" and really mean it.

3. Work Out

I know. Exercising is the last thing you feel like doing. But even a good walk, rain or shine, will take the edge off your hormone-induced misery.

4. Don't Binge

If your normal reaction to stress is wolfing down a bag of Oreos, try not to. The sugar rush—and the post-binge guilt—will just make you feel worse about everything. Trust me on this one: I've been there more times than I would like to admit!

5. Treat Yourself

Do something to take care of yourself: Go for a custom-designed "ahhh moment." Give yourself a facial, take a warm bubble bath (hot water can hurt the baby), shop online for a cute maternity dress that doesn't make you feel like a cow, or read a page-turning novel. Anything you can do to nurture yourself will boost your spirits.

6. Talk to Your Doc

He or she has probably seen every type of pregnancy-induced lunacy known to womankind. Your physician won't respond by saying "My, aren't we unstable!" with a shocked look in her eye. (If she does, switch doctors.)

7. Don't Flog Yourself for Being Emotional

Early on, just tell yourself that you're going to be extra wacky for the next seven months and that you deserve a humdinger of a bawl once in a while (or twice a day). So go ahead and rack up those frequent cryer miles. You'll feel better if you don't fight it.

8. Avoid Movies, Television Shows, and Books that You Know to be Tearjerkers

Let's face it, your tears don't need jerking. If you know that a certain chick flick is known to cause truck drivers to weep uncontrollably (such as *Beaches,* just to name an oldie-but-goodie) just say no. Stick to funny movies, sitcoms, and books. (Paul Reiser's *Babyhood* is laugh-out-loud funny, and you're already preoccupied with the subject anyway.)

9. Last but Not Least, Cling to the Rock

Jesus alone can soothe your ruffled emotions and provide you with a place of true security and comfort. After all, you have this promise: "Come near to God and he will come near to you" (James 4:8). Read the Psalms, and you will be struck by how accurately they give voice to your emotional ups and downs. King David never fails to amaze me with the magnitude of his feelings; he simply seethed with them. The man never met an emotion he didn't embrace, and none of them was mild. When he was happy, he was exultant, bouncing off the ceiling and carrying on so much that his wife told him to cut it out. (He didn't.) But when he was sad or worried or lonely, the guy who came up with "miry pit" to describe his blues was flattened at rock bottom. Sound familiar? The best part of reading David's journal of ups and downs is that they ultimately point to God as the source of strength and security.

Leslie Brandt, in his book *Psalms Now*, has written this moving paraphrase of a portion of Psalm 32:

> You are, O God, a place of refuge;
> You do enable me to face my problems
> You do keep me from being destroyed by them.
> Even within the darkness about us,
> In the midst of life's turmoil,
> One can often hear the voice of God:
> "Even these things serve a purpose in your life.
> Don't sell them short,
> For they may be steps along my path for you."[6]

What to Do This Month

☐ To doula or not to doula? Now is the time to hire a doula, a specialized pregnancy professional who will help you, answer your questions, and be an invaluable labor coach for you. Ask your doctor's opinion, research doulas online, and ask friends who have had doulas about the pros and cons of having such a partner.

☐ Now is also a good time to decide whether you want a midwife, a nurse-midwife, an ob-gyn, or a general doctor to be your medical partner throughout your term, labor, and delivery.

☐ Decide which hospital you want to deliver at (unless you are opting for a home birth) and make sure your insurance carrier covers your choice. Notify your carrier now that you are pregnant. Some health plans won't cover some or all of your prenatal care, labor, and delivery unless you let them know early on that you are expecting. This info is usually in the fine print of your insurance handbook, but it's worth checking just to make sure. The last thing you need is to be denied coverage!

☐ Consult your doctor about beginning an energy-boosting fitness program or adapting your existing exercise routine to carry you through your pregnancy. (More on exercise in chapter 5.)

☐ Journal idea: Tell Baby all about your bouts with morning sickness. You won't remember in ten years that the sight of hot dogs made you violently ill. Besides, by then it should be good for a laugh.

Dear Baby,

We've come to the twelve-week mark together, and I for one am quite relieved. Of course, I know that something could happen to you during the next twenty-eight weeks, but the chances are a whole lot slimmer than they were. I have a good feeling that you and I are in this for the long haul.

My friend Jane just told me she is pregnant too, and this time we are only a week apart in due dates. It's fun to have a buddy to go through this with again. She can completely relate to all the drama and craziness and loop-de-loops. To be able to call someone and say, "Okay, my pants don't fit, and I'm only three months along" and then have her respond with empathy (not, "It's all for a good cause, blah, blah, blah...") is priceless.

Your big brother, Jonah, and Jane's daughter, Avery, are only a month apart, and it's been such fun to watch them grow up and play together. I know this little one and you will also be grand pals. (You're thinking, "Gee whiz, Ma. I'm only a fetus here, and you're already picking my friends!")

Anyway, I think the morning sickness might be subsiding a wee bit now. Maybe. And they say that in a couple of weeks my energy will be back, which means you and I will once again be hitting the gym. (I have been trying to go, but once or twice a week probably isn't doing much for either of us.) This is a fabulous adventure we're on here, sweet child. I'm so glad you're mine.

Love,
Mama

Mood Swings, the Munchies, and (Decaf) Mochas

This particular fun patch of your couplehood presents some of the juiciest, trickiest, and most explosive minefields that you will encounter in your linked together little lives. Never again is a loving husband's ability to tap-dance, turn the other cheek, and "just walk away" put more relentlessly to the test.

—PAUL REISER, *Babyhood*

Snapshot! "Mommy, *wow!* I'm a fetus now!" Yup, by eight weeks, your little squirt will have graduated from embryo to fetus. By the end of the first trimester, Baby is 2-1/2 to 3-inches long and is fully formed. He or she has begun swallowing and kicking. Between weeks twelve and fourteen, your little one will grow by leaps and bounds between three and four inches. Organs and muscles have formed and are beginning to function. Baby is growing bones (drink lots of milk!), fingernails, and toenails and—how cute is this?—is sprouting tiny buds in its gums for a future gap-toothed grin.

Your Guy and You: Navigating the Mood Swings

When Becky was pregnant, she remembers well how the hormonal fluctuations played with both her head and her relationship with her mate Rudy.

"One minute I would be all dreamy over him, thinking things like, 'He still looks as great as he did when we first started dating, maybe even better.' Then the next thing you know, I would be really mad at him over nothing or worried that he had lost his feelings for me. I once called my sister, crying, to tell her that I was sure Rudy didn't love me anymore because he didn't take out the garbage."

Mood swings—you know: anxiety, ambivalence, stress, paranoia, a short fuse—can wreak havoc on that most important relationship with your main man. As Becky said, at times you may feel downright mushy about this fabulous human being with whom you've created a child. What can be—and is widely thought to be by those who have never been with child—an idyllic time of husband and wife knitting booties and hearts in a cohesive, welcoming unit of impending parenthood can also be nine months of hormone- and stress-induced fights and miscues.

 What a Guy

"Oddly enough, Ray and I didn't fight too much during my pregnancies. I think it's partly due to his ability to absorb a bunch of my weirdness without getting back at me and partly due to my knowledge that he wasn't going to respond to my nasty remarks. This last time, though, he did tell me that I was getting psychotic on him."

—Ann

Personally, I think Paul Anka actually wrote his tune "Having My Baby" only partly to express his joy at becoming a father. More likely he was trying to get in his wife's good graces again after committing some sort of felony, like folding the socks wrong or not passing the ketchup in ten seconds or less.

Anita confesses that her marriage was strained to the breaking point during each of her three pregnancies. She felt an overwhelming sense of paranoia that her husband was having an affair, so much so that she became furious when he came home from a fishing weekend with no fish. "I said all kinds of nasty, insinuating things like 'You don't even like fishing.' Stuff like that." Anita's husband was so frustrated and desperate that he even suggested she hire a private investigator to follow him around.

I for one would never think that my own hubby, Doyle, was having an affair if he said he was going fishing. In fact, he does have mistresses I have to compete with: bass, walleye, brook trout, catfish—you get the picture. But I have felt those weird, uneasy doubts that pop up with no warning. And I have definitely experienced flashes of temper, instant fingernails-on-a-chalkboard irritability, and inexplicable tears. I think most of you know of what I speak by now. Sometimes you're not exactly yourself, and sometimes it shows.

Take, for example, my now famous "You don't know where the towels are!" freak-out session early in my second pregnancy. First let me say that Doyle is truly a phenomenal man when it comes to helping around the house. If I am running on a tight deadline, he will drop everything after work and take over dinner, run herd on Jonah, and basically keep the house quiet until whatever I am working on is done. That being said, I was, at the time I promised to tell you about, irritated that the house was in shambles and that he didn't seem to care. While we were eating dinner one night, he left the table to wipe up a spill. He picked up a dishtowel that lay on the counter instead of getting a clean one out of the kitchen drawer. This is where it gets strange (cue up music from *The Twilight Zone*): All I could think was, *He is so utterly unconcerned about this house and how it looks he doesn't even know where the clean towels are!* Neon "tilt" lights flashed. Sparks flew. Smoke billowed. I began to cry, and hot tears streamed down my face as I screeched bloody murder about standards and neglect and towel storage policies. The poor man was stunned. The look on his face was pure deer-in-the-headlights. I rushed upstairs in a maelstrom of righteous indignation. I huffed and I puffed—until about five minutes later when I felt like the biggest buffoon the world had ever encountered. Did I go downstairs, embrace my maligned husband, and apologize ever so sweetly? Not a chance. Like a jerk, I marinated in my pride for a good long while until I realized I had no option whatsoever but to say I was sorry. I apologized a lot during my pregnancies, and chances are you will too.

The first order of business is to talk about this alien life force that has taken your hormones hostage and turned you into Cruella De Vil. The more you can express your concerns, the better your mate will understand you and hopefully cut you some slack. Be as open as you can about feeling paranoid, anxious, sad, irritable, or, if you're lucky enough to have the "deluxe" version of pregnancy lunacy, all of the above. The late Jean Lush, whose pioneering writings on emotions illuminated for countless women the reality of their hormonal upsets, writes about this in her book *Women and Stress:* "Women, do yourselves a favor. Inform your husbands and older children about [emotional phases in one's hormonal cycle] so they know what to expect. They are likely to think you're going crazy…if they don't understand what's happening in your body. It will be much easier for them to tolerate your mood swings if they are informed."[1]

Slowing Swings

Mood swings tend to be most conspicuous in the first twelve weeks of pregnancy. The emotional tilt-a-whirl should calm down as your body gets used to the progesterone rush.

Whenever you can, debrief and defuse. If you can catch yourself before you explode, hie thyself away from there—and quick. A change of scenery, a few deep breaths, and a prayer may help you swerve away from an emotional crash. Try to get some time alone. Even a fifteen-minute shower will make you feel more in control and less likely to take out your baffling emotions on your husband. Writing down your crazy feelings in a journal or on your computer will help you objectify them and make them less volatile. If your mood doesn't improve, or if you suspect more drastic measures are in order, Jean Lush suggests trying a quick release of energy she calls the defusing method. "Defusing is literally keeping a bomb from exploding, or quenching a fire before it burns out of control," she writes in *Emotional Phases of a Woman's Life*. "You can defuse tension by weeding the garden, running, swimming, or doing any intense activity that leaves you physically tired."[2]

Always, the best course of action is spiritual. Pour out your frustrations, anxieties, confusions, guilt—every sloppy, prickly, nonsensical feeling—to your heavenly Father. Ask Him to help you gain command of your emotions and to give you the courage to ask for forgiveness...again. Pray for healing in your emotions and for Him to somehow, through all the ups and downs, knit you and your mate closer together. Once you've prayed it through and (if need be) made things right with your husband, you won't believe how much better you'll feel. I am amazed that God can transform a potentially poisonous thing like a hormone fight into a deepened closeness, a renewed alliance that is stronger than ever.

So if you're just dying to know, yes, Doyle did forgive me, being the gracious guy that he is. And he also knows exactly where the towels are. In fact, he always did.

Eating for Two
(Or One Grown Woman and One Tiny Human the Size of a Lima Bean)

Cooked dried beans. Canned sardines. Kale. Brewer's yeast. Yum yum! Just a cursory reading of almost any guide to pregnant eating will encourage you to somehow work these wonder foods into your diet. Having never knowingly imbibed brewer's yeast, but having personally researched several articles on nutrition, I am always amazed at how seriously impractical many suggested diets are. Not only do these experts propose that you need shredded cabbage for vitamin C or canned salmon for calcium (haven't

"How Can Hubby and I Share This Experience?"

"With all the hormonal weirdness and everything else I'm facing, what can I do to turn my pregnancy into a time for my husband and me to get closer, not further apart?" —MARRIED IN MINNESOTA

Dear Married,

The answer to your question will probably be as unique as your guy himself. I can offer a few suggestions for you, but I suspect whether it works will depend on what Daddy needs as much as on what you need.

For example, my husband hates to read, so leaving interesting highlighted pages around the house for him to peruse wasn't a great idea. Instead I made extra effort to wake up when he did and give him baby updates over coffee before he went to work. I usually climbed back into bed afterward! A friend of mind whose other half is *not* a morning person made similar plans to go to bed at the same time he did so there was time for talk before sleep—no small feat considering how early she wanted to hit the sack! Identify and protect those times that tend to be best for you and your husband to have some focused conversations. Nap around them so that you are fully present and accounted for during your together time.

Keeping my husband involved in the pregnancy in ways that were really meaningful to *him* helped too. He was far less interested in settling on a nursery theme than I was, so forcing him to give me opinions when it was clear he didn't really care or dragging him on lengthy journeys to the crafts or paint and wallpaper stores just made life stressful for both of us. I had to set aside some of my expectations that my entire pregnancy would be as mesmerizing and magical for him as it was for me. Imagine my surprise when I mentioned in passing that I might use the laundry room as a diaper-changing station and he, a real practical handyman, completely reorganized it, surprising me with new shelves, cubbyholes, and a changing table. He even went out and bought newborn diapers and a Diaper Genie. Having a crib or stroller to assemble, or a car seat to install, thrilled him just as much as my nursery-decorating efforts thrilled me. I made a habit of leaving these types of projects for him even if they were simple enough for me to tackle on my own.

Another friend of mine whose guy is a real finance freak spent most of their first pregnancy bent over a calculator. While at first this annoyed his laid-back wife, she found that indulging his fetish for cost-comparison shopping trips, having him keep his eye open for sales, involving him in purchasing decisions, and buying what she could at garage sales and consignment or thrift shops helped ease *his* stress, which meant more peace in general for both of them.

On another baby matter, my family has the somewhat odd tradition of having Dad pick Baby's first name while Mom picks the middle one. Before you say "no way," let me clarify that it isn't exactly a dictatorship. My husband picked a few doozies, and I *quickly* said, "no way." But for the most part I stepped aside and let him pick something he truly liked, then I picked a middle name that matched. While the first names we settled on might not have been my first choices, I can tell you without hesitation that now I can't imagine our children being named anything else.

As for my emotions, that's a tricky storm to ride. It was easier with my second pregnancy than my first to tell when the roller coaster was about to take a dip, but it was easier with my first than my second to temporarily remove myself from the scene. If it's your first pregnancy, hie thyself away to a bathroom, bedroom, coffee shop, or gym when the mood swings hit. If it's your second, ask your guy to help you out when he can (and if he still vividly remembers your first pregnancy, he'll likely be willing!) My second pregnancy turned out to be a terrific time of bonding for my husband and firstborn. They had regular daddy-daughter time while I napped (or flipped out). And although I wouldn't have expected it, their stronger relationship brought a new dimension to our own as well.

—MICHELLE GLEICHMANN, MOTHER OF ADDIE, 5, AND CALEB, 1

these people heard of oranges and milk, for Pete's sake?), they also prescribe a hard-to-interpret metric quota. I don't know about you, but after washing and shredding the cabbage, the last thing I want to do is measure how many micrograms I've got in the cup.

Let's keep it simple. Eating for two shouldn't be rocket science, just healthful, tasty, and fun. Upon finding out that they are pregnant, many women suddenly undergo a metamorphosis. Once the Patron Saint of Pizza, the newly p.g. gal turns into the Goddess of Green, spurning all her junky favorites for a new regimen of organic kale and free-range chicken. Especially if this is your first pregnancy, you may find yourself scrutinizing every morsel of food you put in your mouth. And that's good because your baby deserves lots of extra consideration. But you don't have to go completely bananas in your quest to eat right for Junior's sake. My ob-gyn, Mary Beth Grey, says: "You don't have to go out on a limb, but you have to think, 'Am I getting enough fruits and vegetables, lean proteins? Am I not eating too much of the same food group?' Your diet doesn't have to go crazy. You just need a good, moderate diet." This is good news for those of us plagued by nausea in the first trimester. It's hard enough to keep down favorite foods, never mind canned sardines.

Though morning sickness may cause you to lose weight during your first trimester, you'll make up for it in the next six months. The old adage "you're eating for two" becomes a license for some to indulge in a calorie free-for-all. But it was a stunning disappointment to me when I learned that I couldn't—in good conscience anyway—scarf down a pan of brownies for breakfast and a stuffed pizza for lunch. In fact, your calorie increase right now should only amount to an extra apple and a glass of skim milk, which to me doesn't sound like very much fun. But it's important to remember the second person is only as big as a Hacky Sack, at most, until Month Six or so. So you don't really need to increase your calorie intake until your second trimester and then do so only about two to three hundred calories per day. Your new energy needs then should only require the equivalent of a turkey and Swiss cheese sandwich.

"Most pregnant women should gain between 25 and 35 pounds," says Dr. Grey. "If you're heavy, we don't mind if you gain as little as 15 pounds, but if you start out thin, we want you to gain 30 to 35. Recent studies show that more weight gain contributes to a good fetal outcome."

Gaining enough weight is vital, but so is not gaining too much. Exorbitant pounds contribute to diabetes, not to mention the post-pregnancy struggle to lose weight. A good rule of thumb is to gain about "a half a pound a week in the first trimester, then one pound for every week afterward," suggests Dr. Grey.

The bottom line: Be balanced in your diet. Boost your intake of good proteins, complex carbohydrates, calcium, and fluids. Avoid the big no-nos, like alcohol, soft cheeses, sushi (except for California rolls, which feature cooked crab), and raw eggs (sorry, that includes cookie dough).

And don't expect your prenatals to compensate for what you're unwilling to do yourself. Though taking them daily is important, these specially formulated vitamins can't compensate for dining out of Styrofoam containers morning, noon, and night. "The prenatal vitamin gives you the basics, but you need other things in your diet to balance it out," says dietician Ruth de Boer-Logi. "There are probably nutrients in foods that pregnant women need that we haven't identified yet, so they aren't in the supplements. Fiber in food is important too, especially because vitamins, fortified with iron, can cause constipation." Prenatals are also known to be stingy on calcium, something you and baby both need for bodacious bones.

The Nifty Nine
Tips for Putting the Best Foods in Your Mouth

1. Go for the Calcium

It's something your body needs anyway, according to the good folks who make Tums. But soon enough you are going to be popping Tums to ward against and alleviate heartburn, so you'll have to look for alternate sources of calcium, just for variety. According to a 1997 study by the Institute of Medicine, you don't actually need to take in much more than the recommended 1,000 milligrams per day. Apparently one of the nifty perks of pregnancy is that your body absorbs calcium better, so you only need to have as much as your nonpregnant pals. Still, most women—pregnant or not—don't get anywhere near this amount, so load up on your favorite yogurt, say cheese often, wear a milk mustache, and gulp down those greens. See, here's the thing: If you don't get enough, your baby will actually burglarize your calcium stores, putting you at risk for bone loss later in life (when you can remind her of this fact and politely suggest she now take you in to care for your every need).

2. Water, Water Everywhere...

And you should be drinking pints of the stuff, or at least eight glasses per day. *Yeah, yeah,* you might be thinking. *I've heard this before.* True, but keep track of how much water you actually drink in a day, and you'll be amazed at how far you fall short, not to mention how many times you visit the ladies' room. Water is essential for developing cells, processing nutrients, and maintaining Baby's blood volume. As for you, my swollen-ankled sister, the more water you drink, the less you retain. This fact is something you will deeply appreciate if you, not unlike Cinderella's step-sisters, are ever unable to jam your size seven tootsie into a size eight shoe (true story, unfortunately). And the bonuses just keep coming: Lotsa water also keeps things moving along nicely in terms of your bowels, if I may be so blunt. When your intestines are having what we might call a jam session...well, this thought alone is worth the price of a bottle of Evian.

3. Get Enough Vitamin C

Your body can't store vitamin C, which means that even if you drank a gallon of OJ on Monday, by Tuesday your C tank is empty. A grapefruit with breakfast, a glass of grape juice for lunch, and a couple of sliced tomatoes with your dinner salad is enough to refuel your supplies. A great way to get plenty of C at once is to drink the new orange juice that contains double the RDA of this good stuff. Vitamin C is an amazing little nutrient because it fights off colds and flus for you and manufactures collagen, which is extremely important for structuring Baby's bones, cartilage, muscle, and blood vessels.

4. Brown is Beautiful

Stick to "brown" cereals and breads and you'll be doing your bod—and Baby's—a great favor. As for cereals, brown doesn't have to be as bad as it sounds. I mean, the stuff my parents eat for breakfast looks like rabbit pellets—I wouldn't choke it down at gunpoint. But a bowl of Cheerios is substantially healthier than shaped cereals that feature colors brighter than anything Sherman Williams can come up with. (Even sugary cereals, though, are fortified, which makes them more nutritious, I must admit, than my favorite bagel and cream cheese.) For all grains, including pastas, rice, and bread, a good rule of thumb is "the browner the better." Switch to whole grains and you'll get double the fiber of white varieties. Remember our brief discussion about irregularity—one of the all-time great euphemisms—and pass up the Wonderbread for some nutty twelve-grain. If you still balk, I have one word for you: hemorrhoids.

5. Pump Up the Iron

Because you're growing a human being, you need to double your iron intake. You need it to make hemoglobin, and during pregnancy, your hemoglobin output has to really rev up to supply Baby with oxygen. Your prenatal, if it's worth its salt, should have plenty of iron. Just in case, though, munch a spinach salad with your prime rib. (What's that? You don't eat red meat? Hmmm. Well, double the spinach salad thing and throw some dried beans in there. That ought to do the trick.)

6. Tell Veggie Tales

You must like at least a couple of vegetables, right? Even I, an eater so picky my friends and family dread having to order a pizza with me (no onions, no peppers, no mushrooms…you get the picture), can happily eat carrots and tomatoes. So get into the habit of eating a salad with dinner. Those bags of prewashed, preshredded salads have revolutionized my life. The ones with carrots, sugar snap peas, and darker greens offer a good chunk of your RDA of vitamin A, and you don't have to chop a thing. So pick the vegetables you like (corn doesn't really count), and then figure out fifty different ways to fix them. By the way, iceberg lettuce is not a vegetable. It's just solid light green water.

7. Snack Smart

You will get the munchies at least a few times a day. Instead of potato chips, go for pretzels and air-popped popcorn. There's the fiber incentive, plus you won't be adding to your fat stores. If you think your thighs are pleasingly plump now, just wait until you've gone through nine months and nine hundred bags of Frito Lay products. Nuts also fit the crunchy/salty niche, but, unlike potato chips, they offer good-for-you fats. Other good munchies: cartons of yogurt, bagels with peanut butter, cubes of low-fat cheese, and apples with healthy fruit dip.

8. Eat When You Are Hungry

Your metabolic rate goes up by 20 percent when you're pregnant, which explains why your tummy is grumbling an hour and a half after lunch. After your first trimester, you will be ravenous much of the time, and when a pregnant woman is hungry, watch out! One of the greatest pleasures of pregnancy is eating, so chow down. It's not supposed to be a free-for-all, but you're not dieting or watching your weight either.

9. Cheat Once in a While

You have a voracious appetite, for goodness sake, so you might as well indulge in a big treat every few days or so. If you've been a good girl and munched your carrot quotient, absorbed so much calcium you're beginning to think your name is Bessie, and gnawed on bread so fibrous you feel like a beaver, it's time to throw caution to the wind, throw open the refrigerator, and devour something decadent. Before conception, I had been envisioning pregnancy as a delightful interlude in which I would spend one-on-one time with my new best friends Ben and Jerry. Knowing what I know now about sound nutrition, I must say that the three of us don't get together as often as I had hoped. Still, half a carton of New York Chocolate Chunk every so often does a world of good.

What About Coffee?

You may quake at the thought of foregoing your morning cup of java while you're pregnant. I did. To be honest, I simply could not wait for the glorious morn, post-pregnancy, when I could freely drink more than one cup to evaporate my A.M. foggies. Fortunately, coffee is allowed—up to a point. But if you are used to an espresso in the morning, a glass of iced tea in the afternoon, and a mocha latte at night, you will need to scale back for the sake of Baby.

"Caffeine crosses the placenta and enters the fetus, where it may affect fetal heart rate and breathing," says Ruth. This is a hard, cold fact, and a sobering one at that. Still, overwhelming evidence points to moderate caffeine intake as being just fine. If only someone could define "moderate." As far as I can tell, most in-the-know types would like for us in-the-condition types to curb our caffeine to two hundred milligrams a day. *Well, wait just a minute,* you might be thinking. *Weren't you just dissing the cabbage shredders and their metric minutiae?* True, I was. But unfortunately, caffeine is measured in milligrams exclusively. Also unfortunate: It's almost impossible to find a food or beverage label that identifies how much caffeine coffee contains. So for your sake I've done some homework and made the handy dandy chart on the next page to help you get a handle on which of your favorite goodies are inundated with the stuff.

Beverage/Food	Serving Size	Caffeine
Diner coffee	8 ounces	350 milligrams
Gourmet coffee	8 ounces	175 milligrams
Brewed coffee	5 ounces	105 to 115 milligrams
Espresso	single	100 milligrams
Cappuccino	single	100 milligrams
Instant coffee	6 ounces	57 milligrams
Decaffeinated coffee	5 ounces	5 milligrams
Brewed tea	6 ounces	20 to 110 milligrams
Iced tea	12 ounces	70 milligrams
Instant tea	7 ounces	30 milligrams
Cola	1 12-ounce can	30 to 56 milligrams
Diet cola	1 12-ounce can	38 to 45 milligrams
Non-cola	1 12-ounce can	54 milligrams
Sprite and 7-Up	1 12-ounce can	0 milligrams
Chocolate	2 ounces	10 to 50 milligrams
Cocoa	1 5-ounce cup	4 milligrams

Research into the effects of drinking more than three or four cups of coffee a day offers both confusing and inconsistent results, so experts don't always agree on how to advise pregnant women. To stay on the safe side, ask your doctor's advice, watch your caffeine intake, and pay attention to insidious caffeine carriers (especially chocolate, colas, and certain medicines) which may pop you right over your limit.

If the people in your universe are anything like the ones in mine were, they will watch you like hawks anyway. Soon after I found out I was pregnant, I was at a church potluck with my friend Margaret, never one to keep her opinions to herself. Just as I was lifting a fabulous looking, gooey and rich chocolate-chip cookie to my mouth, she had a fit: "Whaddya think you're doing?" she squawked in her best New Jersey accent. "You're pregnant! You can't have chocolate!" I find her watchdog reaction to be somewhat typical.

When you're pregnant, the whole world appoints itself your guardian, and everyone will surely feel free to at least glare meaningfully should you be seen indulging in some activity (jumping on a trampoline, jogging, mowing the lawn) or food item they deem unsuitable. You'll see what I mean the first time you belly up to the Starbucks counter and order a decaf caramel latte because only the person who took your order knows it's decaf. The rest of the patrons will give you the hairy eyeball in a manner that suggests you are actually freebasing street drugs.

 Fact or Fable?

You're laying low on the joe, but you should also be watching what kinds of herbal teas you're drinking. Remember, herbs can be potent and medicinal. Red raspberry tea has been blamed for causing early labor. An old wives' tale? Maybe. Ask your doctor and find out for sure.

So what does caffeine actually do to your baby? Well, nothing too heinous, but nothing positive either. It's a stimulant, which boosts your heart rate and metabolism, a stress to Baby. Keep in mind, though, that climbing a big flight of stairs will do the same thing. But while *unremitting* stress isn't healthy, *brief* bouts of fetal stress, such as what your baby would feel after you drink a cup of coffee, won't cause him any harm.

I'm not going to lecture you any further about the possible drawbacks of coffee drinking. Goodness knows your friends and relatives will be glad to tell you all about its various ill effects, all the while sipping their grande cappuccinos. If you want to cut back on caffeine, you may find your taste buds making the way easier. Even I, a person as fond as anyone of her morning cuppa, found coffee a bit sickening during those morning sickness days. But if your yen for Costa Rican supreme returns—as it did to me—try the following:

- Switch to tea, which has substantially less caffeine and steep your teabag for only a minute or two.

- Mix up or buy some half-and-half coffee blends. You may not even miss the 50 percent caffeine.
- Experiment with instant or, better yet, flavored instant coffee.
- Not all soda pop contains the same amount of caffeine. Switch to Diet Rite, with the lowest: 35 milligrams. It has only half the caffeine of Jolt cola, and you'll soon get used to the taste.

The Pickles and Ice Cream Hall of Fame

Cravings—Paul Reiser calls them "prenatal takeout" orders—are an incontrovertible rite of passage for pregnant women. In fact, many women are crestfallen when they don't actually experience any out-of-the-ordinary appetites. But for those of us who do, the absolute fits of longing for a particular food will not soon be forgotten. Cravings don't have to be weird (although of course it makes for a better story at parties and with the grandkids); they just have to seize your body and mind with the unyielding wish to devour a certain something.

One day I just *had* to have sesame chicken, no ifs, ands, or buts about it. I mean, every cell in my body was blitzkrieged with ardor for sesame chicken. Unfortunately, my oblivious husband picked that day to be late from work, which meant that, with every moment the clock ticked, my voraciousness ballooned. I couldn't just leave my two-year-old at home while I chased that chicken, and it seemed like a good idea to wait so we could all go out to eat as a family. (At that point, my craving was still low enough on the Richter scale that I *cared* if my husband came home to an empty house and no food.) I tore through the house trying to find that Chinese takeout menu which I could have sworn said "delivery." Alas, it was gone, and I couldn't remember the name of the restaurant. Arrrgh! Things were getting worse by the second! Finally I grabbed my son and went to wait for his dad out on the sidewalk. You know how they say a watched pot never boils? I'm here to tell you that a watched-for vehicle— especially one that's supposed to transport a pregnant woman with cravings to the delicacy of her dreams—never materializes. (And meanwhile Doyle, completely unaware of his wife's Szechwan Seizure, was merrily tooling down the highway, *going the speed limit.* The nerve! Can you believe it?)

To say I began frothing at the mouth would be an exaggeration, but my neighbor Mandy was somewhat alarmed by my wild-eyed, rather frantic self. Jonah began eyeballing me with some concern, thinking to himself that Mommy was three fries short of a Happy Meal. Finally, I could take no more. I ran into the house, scribbled a note about our whereabouts, and made a mad dash for Seoul Garden.

Read of the Month (and Beyond)

Subscribe to *Fit Pregnancy* magazine, my fave, for great tips on eating right, exercising, and coping with all other aspects of pregnancy. You don't have to be a big workout fiend to benefit, and the writing is always fresh and sometimes funny. A pregnant friend told me not long ago that, out of the deluge of magazines available for expectant moms, this was the one she read cover to cover. I agree wholeheartedly!

You'll think I'm exaggerating unless, of course, you've been there. But, truthfully, cravings can capsize a normally calm and reasonable woman at any time of the day or night.

John remembers being awakened at four in the morning by his wife, Pam, who had the urge for a Denny's Grand Slam breakfast. Certainly, what happened next should prequalify John for sainthood: He roused his slumbering self out of bed, got dressed, and drove his wife to Denny's, a half-hour away by car. As they sat in Denny's, with the light of the morning sun still another hour or so away, John was now fully awake. When the eggs and hash browns and sausages arrived, though, Pam took one bite and decided she really wasn't in the mood for a Grand Slam after all. John's reaction? (You may want to highlight this section and casually leave it lying around the house.) He took it in stride, saying, "Well, she was pregnant. I gotta do my part too." They went on to have three kids.

The moral of the story is that cravings can be very fickle business. And a woman possessed thereof may not be exactly in her right mind. Here are some of the more unusual cravings I've heard of:

- Cherry pie filling straight out of the can
- Green beans straight out of the can

 Testing One, Two, Three (Four, Five...)

All that poking and prodding your physician is doing to you is for a great cause. Here are some of the tests you can expect as a matter of course:

- *Right-off-the-bat lab stuff:* Blood tests determine your blood type and screen for a number of problems, including anemia. A pap smear rules out cervical cancer.

- *Once-a-checkup:* Get used to peeing in a cup. Your doc will test your urine each month for protein and sugar levels.

- *Triple test:* Between fifteen and twenty-two weeks, your doc will probably suggest you have your blood tested for higher-than-normal levels of certain hormones, which may indicate your risk of Down's syndrome or neural tube defects. Many women choose not to have this test because false positives are both common and incredibly nerve-wracking.

- *Glucose screening:* Between twenty-four and twenty-eight weeks, you'll get to gulp down this sickly-sweet glucose drink

- Stewed tomatoes straight out of the can (Hmmm, could there be a theme here?)
- Tuna and watermelon, in bed, in the middle of the night
- Greek olives right out of the container, at the grocery store, prior to checkout. Or check out this olive edition: "Four days before I had any inkling I was pregnant at all, I finished off the green olives (with pimientos) and drank all the juice," says Becky, 32. "I think I even licked the lid. That's pregnancy."
- Chalk

and then have your blood drawn. It's not only gross, but it may make you dizzy, too. This test assesses your risk for gestational diabetes. Make sure you drink the stuff chilled (and maybe even don't breathe to take the edge off the foulness).

- *Group B strep:* Between thirty-five and thirty-seven weeks, when you've seen so much of your doctor you're on the verge of calling him "Uncle Monty," the time will come for him to take a culture from your vagina to test for Group B streptococcus, a potentially dangerous bacteria that can be passed on to your baby during delivery. If it comes back positive, your doctor will treat you with antibiotics.

- *Other, more complicated tests*—such as amniocentesis, chorionic villus sampling (CVS), non-stress test—may also arise depending on how your pregnancy is going, your age, your family medical history, and so on. You need to be calm, cool, and collected, not to mention informed. So don't be shy about asking your doctor any and all questions you may have about any test, routine or otherwise!

- Houseplant soil (I kid you not. This woman, who is a distant relative, craved earth so badly she would scoop up little handfuls of the stuff at people's homes when the hosts left the room. I would love to be able to tell you that she experienced bizarre side effects from this, such as an African violet growing out her ear, but it simply wouldn't be true. As it is, the truth is stranger than anything I could make up!)
- Lemons ("I craved lemons to the point where I had to have them on everything—every salad, everything," actress Amy Yasbeek told *In Style* magazine. I made my husband [actor John Ritter] sick; he said it was like eating Pledge. I guess I just couldn't get enough vitamin C. Luckily, my teeth didn't fall out.")
- Mineral supplements ("My mom had these natural mineral supplement pills. I'd rip open the capsule and eat it," model Tuesday Cook told *Fit Pregnancy* magazine. "I was craving it so bad I would suck on it and grit it in my teeth. My doctor was like, 'Um, okay.'"[3])

What to Do This Month

☐ Talk to your doctor about prenatal tests. (See the related sidebar in this chapter.)

☐ If your clothes are starting to get a tad snug, upgrade and buy a few key pieces in bigger sizes and with stretchy waistbands. Hit up your previously pregnant friends for some loaners.

☐ Research good nutrition and plan some good-for-you, good-to-eat meals.

☐ Take your husband out for a date to his favorite Mongolian BBQ, or fix a wonderful, romantic dinner for two. Make sure he feels as if he's included in this pregnancy, and let him know how thrilled you are to be starting (or continuing) a family with him. Investing in your marriage is crucial, especially now that a munchkin will soon be in the picture. More on this in chapter 5.

☐ Tell! Break the news to anyone and everyone if you haven't already. Make sure to tell the key players—your parents and in-laws, sibs, best friends, boss—before telling the rest of the world.

☐ Journal idea: Tell Baby how you chose to break the news to Grandma, Grandpa, and other close family members, and how they responded to the news.

Dear Baby,

Here we are at sixteen weeks, showing our united front to the world! A couple of weeks ago, I felt you fluttering around inside me for the first time. I once heard the first movements described as "butterfly flutters," which of course makes me think of that song "Butterfly Kisses." That tune is about a girl and her daddy, and even though we have a boy and you could very well be a boy too, it still makes me glassy-eyed whenever I hear it. (By the time you can read this, you will know that "glassy-eyed" is a reference to your Oma, who uses that phrase instead of "misty-eyed." Daddy and I think it is hilarious because "glassy-eyed" is supposed to mean someone is drunk, and Oma's firm motto in life has been "Lips that touch wine will never touch mine." Anyway, it's sort of one of those inside, family jokes that no one else thinks is very humorous. You have to know the people involved, you know?)

Anyway, I digress, as usual. Feeling you inside me is amazing, and now that I have more pep in my step I am really enjoying carrying you around. I almost forgot: Great news, Babe! You are going to have a cousin your very own age, just like Daddy has his cousin Brenda, and I have my cousin Rick, and Jonah has Amanda. Uncle Dan and Aunt Tina announced they are having a baby in February, just six weeks after you arrive! I can't wait to get you and your cousin together.

Love,
Mama

Month Four

Glowing, Growing, and Good, Good, Good Vibrations

Oh yes, you shaped me first inside, then out;
you formed me in my mother's womb.
I thank you, High God—you're breathtaking!
Body and soul, I am marvelously made!
I worship in adoration—what a creation!
You know me inside and out,
you know every bone in my body;
You know exactly how I was made, bit by bit,
how I was sculpted from nothing into something.
Like an open book, you watched me grow from conception to birth;
all the stages of my life were spread out before you,
The days of my life all prepared
before I'd even lived one day.

—PSALM 139:13-16, MSG

Snapshot! This month you can call your baby "Jughead" for a silly little nickname because your baby's head is huge in comparison to his body. He is covered with a layer of thick, downy hair called lanugo. You may have already heard the magical sounds of his heartbeat. Your baby's eyebrows and hair have begun to grow (hmmm…wonder what color his hair will be), and he's getting downright active now, incorporating sleeping, waking, kicking, swallowing, and even peeing into his daily routine. At the very end of this month, you may experience the most amazing thing: quickening, the name for those first butterfly-wing flutters. Don't worry if you don't. There's a wide range of time when moms first feel baby move.

The Good, the Bad, and the Ugly:
The Straight Story on How Pregnancy Will Affect Your Body

I, like hundreds of thousands of modern women, get the Victoria's Secret catalog. I don't recall signing up for it, but there it is, in my mailbox three times a week—at least. You won't believe me when I tell you that the reason I don't cancel it is because I love their flannel pajamas, but it's true. I don't know how long you have been married, but if it's more than a couple of years, you know what I'm talking about. As a newlywed, my motto for lingerie was "easy on, easy off, looks good on the floor." After nine years of wedded bliss, however, the motto has been shortened to "easy on." Period.

And my definition of *lingerie* has certainly changed as well. The silky wee slips of fabric I used to wear are now decomposing in my drawer from disuse. Now it's all about comfort—and that explains my growing collection of polar bear pajamas.

So back to the catalog girls and their gravity-defying physiques (personally, I think Victoria does have a secret: duct tape). WHEN PREGNANT, DO NOT, I REPEAT, DO NOT FLIP THROUGH THIS OR ANY OTHER LINGERIE, UNDERWEAR, OR BATHING SUIT CATALOG! Take the thing and send it straight to recycling. The last thing you need to do is dwell on the fact that your body does not measure up to these Amazon ladies, who are surely genetic anomalies, each one. I tried telling myself that the chicks in these publications have never had children, until I found out one of their main models—Stephanie Seymour—has at least three.

Few women emerge from pregnancy without having at least a few pangs about their changing appearance. Even if you are over the moon about being in the family way, you may from time to time experience a few moments of the uglies. After all, not only does your uterus grow 500 times its normal size (which means your belly is not far behind), but your entire body—head to toe—changes. I won't lie: Some of the changes are not pretty. Some will make you feel utterly freakish. Fortunately, most of the changes are temporary. In the meantime, the following is a heads-up on the coming bodily modifications—or mutations, as you might think of them—plus ways to downplay the bad and play up the good.

 ## Is It Safe to Color Your Hair While You're Pregnant?

The jury is still out on this question, although many experts, including the American College of Obstetrics and Gynecology (ACOG), give pregnant women the green light. While no one has enough information to promise that using chemical dyes is totally safe, it's also true that no one has conclusive data showing that dyes can cause birth defects.

From Rapunzel to Rogaine. This is one of those good news/bad news deals. The good news is your hair will grow like crazy. So will your nails. Between revved-up circulation, those busy pregnancy hormones, and your powerful prenatal vitamins, your skin cells (and thus follicles) will be gorged with nutrition, causing the Rapunzel Effect. The bad news is that your hair will get thicker, which may cause it to feel droopy and dull. The really bad news: You might start growing hair in alarming places, like your chin, your back (wince), and your belly (wince, wince). I'm not saying it will happen—it probably won't—but be prepared and try to remember that this, too, shall pass. In fact, after the baby is born your hair will probably fall right out. (Well, you will probably shed about five times as much hair as usual, which is still not a cheery thought. By then, though, you will be so consumed with Baby that you won't even notice. Probably.)

Glowing skin (and otherwise). Here's one category where I'll share the bad news first (unfortunately the bad news comes in bulk this time), and then I'll try to revive your flagging spirits with a pep talk about That Glow. Sit down, my friend, because this litany of possible skin conditions will make you dizzy. Do you break out before your period? Count on breaking out even more during your pregnancy. A zit here and there won't seem too bad, though, next to blotches caused by extra melatonin. And the blotches will pale in comparison to spider veins, thanks to dilating blood vessels, and moles, courtesy of—what else?—hormones. Then there is the possibility of rashes, linea nigra (a dark line splitting your belly in half), and even skin tags (dry, leathery flaps that take up residence in either visible or high-friction areas of your body like your neck and underarms). Make a pact with yourself here and now not to look too closely at your neck or underarms. (Instruct mate to do same.) Well, I warned you. It's bad. But all of this horrifying information should be weighed against the fact that your skin is absolutely in the pink, radiating so prettily due to high estrogen levels that no one—I'm sure—will even notice a few blotches, moles, or the odd dry leathery flap.

Smile... It kills me that all those commercials about mouthwash and toothpaste always refer to "the gum disease gingivitis," as if we could get it mixed up with the "epiglottis disease gingivitis" or something. That off my chest, apparently there is also a pregnancy variety of the gum disease called you-know-what. Not only do most pregnant women experience bleeding and puffy gums, but we are ten times more likely to get cavities. So brush and floss like a madwoman. (And tell your dentist that you're pregnant—skip those X-rays.)

Spider (vein) woman. Depending on your own personal genetic pool, you may or may not suddenly sprout bluish veins on your legs, and they may or may not be the bulging variety. Credit these beauties to extra blood flow and the pressure of your growing belly, which causes blood and fluid to pool in your lower body. The first time I noticed a varicose vein meandering down the back of my leg, I was truly miffed. The good news is that most of your blue visitors will leave a few months after you give birth. For now, drink a lot of fluids, kick back with your feet up at least as high as your waist a couple times a day, and try maternity hose. (You'll have to get past the words "compression" and "support," which make it sound as if you're about 100. What's next for us—the Craftmatic Adjustable Bed?)

 ## You May Now Move About the Country

High-school reunion? College roommate's wedding? Business trip? Your second trimester is prime time for traveling, because you're not sick and nappy all the time, nor are you huge and unwieldy. For optimum success, take some time and plan for any eventuality. Schedule extra time for delays, wear loose clothing, pack portable snacks, and get up and stretch if you've been sitting too long. Most of all, relax and have a ball, because once the bambino arrives, your traveling days are finito—for a few months anyway.

Doughy digits. If this is your first pregnancy, you might have a hard time believing that your feet can actually grow. Guess what: For the first time since you were oh, fifteen or so, your feet will enlarge. First of all, there is the swelling caused by water retention. Then there is the possibility that you could actually put fat on your feet if you gain too much weight. But the most bizarre cause of your doughy digits is actually the hormone relaxin, which is designed to soften your pelvis bones for labor. This hormone can also cause the bones in your feet to spread, which often leads to permanent jumps in foot size. It's true. I have a closet full of size-seven shoes I'll never wear again. There's a 50 percent chance you'll luck

out and your tootsies will return to their normal size. There's also a 50 percent chance they won't.

Two things to keep in mind as you consider these changes: One, how
you look is all in the eye of the beholder. Many people consider pregnant
women to be gloriously beautiful and their blossoming bodies to be astonishing, awe-inspiring testimonies to divine creativity. Certainly never again
will friends, kin, and strangers consider a potbelly to be "adorable," "cute,"
or "sweet." Recently at a family gathering, my kid brother, newly sensi-
tized by his wife's own pregnancy, stunned me with a compliment. "You
know what," he said, "you look really good when you're pregnant." He
even asked some innocent bystanders, "Doesn't she look great?" Considering this is the same person who once ridiculed me for having ears like a
Vulcan, I was quite agog. But if my brother can appreciate the peerless
charm of pregnancy, chances are excellent that lots of other people do too.

Second, and more vital, beauty isn't everything. It's not even at all
important in the big scheme of things. I mean, yes, an enormous belly,
dry leathery skin tags, and big, puffy feet do sort of conjure up the image
of an elephant, but so what? As my friend Jane says, pregnancy is a time to
"think about the world's standards of how you look, how it's impossible to
look that way, and how they're totally different from God's standards."

Jane is right. At times when we can't possibly "compete" in the looks
department, we're forced to think more about the things that truly matter.
Your most treasured relationships—with God, with your husband, and
with this unbelievably wonderful miracle growing inside you—should be
your focus. Honestly, living as we do in our looks-obsessed world, this
nine-month opportunity to take a breather from playing "mirror, mirror
on the wall" can be downright refreshing. In this season of weight gain,
blotches, and bleeding gums, you can grow by leaps and bounds as a
person! Your character can become more solid! Your wisdom can deepen!
Your appreciation for the infinite and profound can expand! And besides,
when you cradle that amazing baby in your arms for the first time, all the
varicose veins in the world won't matter one bit.

Can You Relate?

From the moment you make them aware of Baby's existence, your family, friends, and complete strangers will relate to you differently. And you will connect with them in a whole new way too.

    Journal to My Grandchild

Kathi Landon, a first-time grandma from Lansing, Michigan, began writing a journal to her unborn grandchild the day she learned her daughter was pregnant. In it she wrote down her hopes and dreams and prayers for the baby, along with favorite Scripture verses. She recorded her feelings the day she found out the baby was a girl; she wrote how certain she was her daughter and son-in-law would be wonderful parents. Topics included her political views, her faith walk, her values, passions, and concerns. By the time baby Zoe was born, Grandma Kathi felt incredibly bonded to her already because she had been devoting such time to thoughts of her granddaughter for so long. Kathi laminated the journal and had it spiral-bound. She then gave it to Zoe the day after she was born. What a phenomenal gift for both Zoe and her grandma!

Your husband, of course, is the key player most invested in this new life you've both had a role in creating. Get ready: Your relationship is about to be transformed. "When you have a baby, you set off an explosion in your marriage," says screenwriter/director Nora Ephron, the film mastermind behind such chick flicks as *Sleepless in Seattle* and *You've Got Mail.* "And when the dust settles, your relationship will be different from what it was. Not better necessarily; not worse, necessarily; just different."[1]

You already know how your pregnancy has shifted and shaped your alliance with your mate. (I covered that in chapters 2 and 3, in case you missed it.) But how will these significant nine months—and your role as mother—change your other relationships? Since you can expect an "explosion" in your marriage, don't be surprised by shake-ups big and small in your connections with the clan and in your friendships of all heights and depths. When those who share your personal orbit become accustomed to you as an actual card-carrying mother, you may be surprised by the rewarding results.

Parents of the Parents

You'll be amazed by how much your appreciation for your mother goes up during your pregnancy.

Juliana remembers the defining moment when her link with her mom was fortified forever. "When I was giving birth to Jonathan, she couldn't come in the room and was sitting in the hallway. For just a few seconds, a nurse had opened the door and my mom and I made eye contact. At that moment, I could truly understand for the first time what it was like for her to be a mother, what she loved about it, and what she loved about her children. Since then I have understood her in a deeper way."

My own mother never experienced pregnancy; my brother and I are both adopted. Still, she has been transfixed by the minutiae of each of my terms like only a grandma-to-be could. And for the first time, I finally got it through my thick skull just how intense and demanding and soul-consuming it was for her to mother me. During my pregnancies, I became downright sappy as I thought about some of the sacrifices my mom made for me. I remember mother-daughter dresses, beautifully hand sewn. I recall a cool hand on my feverish forehead, not to mention hot lunches on freezing Manitoba days. I think about the time my mom cried with me through an angst-ridden night after what's-his-name broke my seventeen-year-old heart. If I had never become a mother, I may still be blithely taking these things for granted.

Your relationship with your dad—or "Grandpa," as he may have taken to calling himself—will likely undergo a similar reevaluation. As you watch your husband's face light up as he watches the ultrasound or frown in worry when you tell him you haven't felt the baby lately, you might catch a glimpse of how much your dad cared about you even before you were born.

When I was pregnant with Jonah, my dad applied himself vigorously to studying the nuances of brain development in infants. All of a sudden he was suggesting that I listen to classical music and urging me to quit drinking coffee. It was sort of touching. (In moderation.)

You might also find yourself more willing to cut your parents some slack. In the past, if you felt a lecture coming on, maybe you let the answering machine take a few calls until you felt it was safe to pick up again. Now you might actually sit through the lecture and learn a thing or two. You might even review your personal history in a less biased light: Okay, so Mom and Dad made no bones about their opinion of that motorcycle-riding-long-haired-gainfully-unemployed-garage-band-boyfriend of yours from 1988, but now that you've grown your own baby girl, you can kind of see their point. (Maybe he *was* a bit skanky, on second thought. Cute, but altogether too wild in retrospect. When you picture your daughter on the back of a Harley—yes, he had a Harley—traveling at warp speed, clutching tightly to the hoodlum's waist—yes, he suddenly *is* a hoodlum—you'll want to call your parents and commend them on their wisdom.)

Of course, the generation gap being what it is, you might experience friction rather than utopia with the folks, especially where differing ideas about pregnancy and child rearing are concerned. Maybe your folks object to the name you've picked out for Baby. (Skip ahead to chapter 6. It's a good idea not to share too much until it's too late.) One grandma-to-be reportedly threatened to disown her future grandchild if her daughter actually used the name proposed. Mom rolled her eyes and named the baby as she wished. Of course that itty-bitty baby melted Granny's heart, and she forgot all about her issue with the name.

Grandparents-to-be are infamous for butting in where they don't technically belong. Their good intentions aside, hearing about how midwives are for hippies, or how mom drank a pot of coffee a day when she was pregnant with you—and look how you turned out!—or that only "women's libbers" combine careers and family can be grinding, to say the least.

In-Law or Outlaw?

"When it comes to moms rating their mother-in-law, just over half (52%) think she is a good influence on their children (vs. 68% who feel that way about their mom). 39% gripe that their mother-in-law doesn't realize how much things have changed since she raised kids, and 55% complain that she gives them too much unwanted advice and/or is critical of how they discipline their kids (make that 60% of those who live nearby)."

—*Child* magazine, May 2001

The stereotype of mothers-in-law is that they are pushy, manipulative, terrifying creatures who baby their grown son within an inch of his life and live to criticize their daughters-in-law's every move. I have heard stories that make me thank God for my own good fortune. I pretty much won the mother-in-law Lotto with Doyle's mom. She's unobtrusive to a fault, wouldn't dream of manipulation, and delivers with the utmost tact any suggestions she might have. I couldn't have designed a better in-law myself.

Certainly, unwanted tips on pregnancy and raising babies are even less welcome when they come from your in-laws. But some pregnant women report that having a baby strengthens family ties with the in-laws, especially the mother-in-law. As Vicki Iovine points out in the *Girlfriend's Guide to Pregnancy,* "Remember, this is a woman who would bite her own arm off to make your little baby more comfortable, OR EVEN BABYSIT IF BEGGED. Even if she doesn't seem all that crazy about you, she will love her son's baby. And if you are a loving mother to her grandchildren, she will probably learn to love you too. Put it this way: If it's ever going to happen, now is the time."[2]

Let's hope your in-laws will be tied with your husband's in-laws for the Gaga Over Baby Award. Anyone who shows the good sense to appreciate the stellar qualities of your offspring merits a few bonus points. Jonah and I once sat behind Jerry Springer on a flight to Canada. Not only did the notorious talk show host not complain about my son's loud, toddler commentary on everything from the peanuts to the clouds to the propellers, but he smiled graciously at us and told me that Jonah was a "real cutie." Not that I've taken to watching his program, mind you, but I've begun to wonder in my weaker moments if Jerry might be just a tad misunderstood.

Try to remember that your parents and your in-laws love your baby, probably second only to your guy and you. Kept at the front of your thinking, this fact will cover a multitude of irritations and potential fall outs (trust me). After all, it's hard to argue with people who think your child is God's gift to the Free World, a baby so appealing, so brilliant and gifted it boggles their minds—and yours.

Friends for All Seasons

One of my favorite things about finding out I am pregnant is calling my girlfriends—scattered from sea to shining sea and north to the Arctic—and making the exciting announcement. My long-distance bill has been notoriously high at these times, but the glee on the other end of the phone is worth every dime. (I love getting those calls, too!)

Breaking the news over lunch is fun, especially when the pal is local. My friend Mary Jo just made my day by announcing that, after over a year of trying to get pregnant, she was indeed with child. There we were, sipping hot drinks, catching up, when she burst out with the splendid news. Despite the fact that we were in a public place, I let out a big gasp, followed by a little shriek, tears, and more gasping. Other diners started to notice my blubbering and carrying on, but I didn't care. The occasion called for disregard of basic restaurant protocol, and I got up and gave my elated buddy a big hug.

Now men break the news differently to their friends. "Hey, did I tell you my wife is pregnant?" is followed by, at most, a grin and a suitable statement of salutation like: "Start saving your money now. Those little rug rats are money pits" or "You'll never fish again, my friend." Rarely do men gasp, shriek, blubber, or, for that matter, hug.

That's why I'm glad I'm a woman. Luckily, most females love pregnancy, especially in others. Sharing such happy news with a dear friend is surely a boon to the soul, but it can also be the beginning of big changes in your relationship. If your friend is also pregnant, you might find yourselves developing a bond for life. Nothing cements a friendship like experiencing pregnancy together. For one thing, you can safely vent, openly air your fears, freely whine, and generally blather on endlessly about the burning topic on both your minds. You can compare notes and share tips.

With others you need to exercise a modicum of courtesy. It's just possible that every single other person you know is not quite as infatuated with your pregnancy as you are. And there are women out there—unbeknownst to you—who've longed for a child yet never conceived. But with a Parallel Pregnant Pal, you can trade off describing, in miniscule detail, every little aspect of gestation.

Friends who have been pregnant come a close second in the sharing stories category. They've been there, done that, so pregnancy is a subject most of them feel comfortable discussing—probably at length. You'll be amazed by how often you'll pick up the phone for a "Did this happen to you?" chat. Plus, these are the pals who will understand completely when you beg off a lunch date because you're sick and exhausted or, later, when Baby has an ear infection.

One note of caution: If there is one thing moms love, it is regaling people with their labor stories. While this is mostly a fun and educational thing, it can also work to your detriment. Especially if you're a first timer, hearing about marathon labors of mind-warping pain can be a little daunting. Yet it's good to prepare yourself for any eventuality, so listening and absorbing these stories can be beneficial. But remember: Just because

Cousin Chatty Cathy used sound effects to recount how badly her perineum tore is no reason to believe you will go through the same thing. Every labor is unique, and yours might be a whole lot easier than hers.

When I became pregnant with Jonah, people suggested that from then on I would have more in common with my friends who were mothers than those who weren't. I didn't want to believe them, because some of my most precious relationships are with single people or those with no kids. But now I believe those people—to a point.

Read of the Month

Don't miss the exhaustive Focus on the Family Complete Book of Baby and Child Care, with primary author Paul C. Reisser, and with a foreword by Dr. James Dobson.

Yes, my other mommy friends and I always have a plethora of stories and quips and advice to share with each other. The topic of childbearing and rearing is ever fresh and interesting. But there are other topics, too. (It used to drive me up a wall, in my Double Income No Kids [DINK] days, to go to a baby shower, or some other gathering of women, and hear about little Bobby's potty training capers and wee Annie's teething issues. Not that I minded cute anecdotes in small doses, but it seemed that the only thing young mothers did was glom onto each other and yak about their precious offspring in infinitesimal detail. Truly, that's not *all* we moms talk about.) Yet trying to maintain and nurture a friendship with someone who can't relate to the most important thing in your life does get tricky sometimes. But it can be done, especially if you are mindful. Cheryl Richardson, in her book *Take Time for Your Life*, talks about being intentional in friendship: "If you long for high quality relationships and deeper connections with others, embrace that desire fully... Many people shy away from taking an active role in community building. They feel it should come 'naturally,' the way it 'used to.' Keep in mind that it's your choice; you can spend your time in dozens of pleasant chats, or you can have meaningful conversations, trustworthy friends, and uplifting relationships. The effort will pay off."[3]

One of my dearest longtime friends is Carla, who has known me since I was fourteen and totally squirrelly. (It must be said she was also quite a loon.) There's a whole bunch of history between us, and it would be a shame to let that slide because I'm a mother and she's not. She and her husband have chosen not to be parents. They live in downtown Ottawa and lead what appears to me to be an exotic life of takeout and travel. I live in a *Leave It to Beaver* neighborhood and lead a life of fish sticks and minivans. But Carla and I still manage to hold lengthy conversations about music, books, politics, our families, and memories of the good old days. She cares about Jonah and sends him thoughtful, creative gifts. He will benefit from growing up knowing his mother's wild and crazy pal—who'd better not, ahem, tell him certain stories from our shared adolescence! Pregnancy and ensuing motherhood did change our friendship, but we got over the inevitable hump and adjusted to this new stage of our relationship.

When you become pregnant, you don't have to lose dear friendships or become someone new and unrecognizable. You're still you, just more bloated and cranky. Hold on to the relationships that feed your soul and give you joy. They will change, true, but with a little sensitivity and mindfulness, the change will all be for the good.

Pregnant Sex: The Nifty Nine Guidelines for "Finishing the Baby"

One of my friend's moms is a vivacious, warm, and wonderful person who mothers in the best possible way all who come into her circle of influence. Through years of basking in her nurturing, I have gleaned highly usable bits of wisdom. Of course, one's ears perk up when the topic of sex is broached, especially by a spiritual and together chick like Mrs. W. One of her most practical, coy, and altogether cheeky little tips is about pregnant sex.

Most people don't believe sex is just for procreating (if it were so, God wouldn't have slipped Song of Solomon into His canon), but Mrs. W had a cure for anyone who thought so. Yes, the sperm and egg have merged successfully, but now you have nine months to, as she says with a wink, "finish

 Sensitivity Training

Endless chatter about children and pregnancy may be merely annoying to some, but for a woman who is infertile, such talk is painful. I was recently at a luncheon when I noticed that *look* in one woman's eyes. She was trying to appear interested but not quite selling it. Oops. She didn't have kids, and the rest of us did. I shut my flapping jaws and tried to think of something non-parenting to say, some way to introduce her into the conversation. Admittedly, this was not easy.

Obviously, the sensitive thing to do is to refrain from talking about your pregnancy around a friend struggling with infertility. Unless she asks, don't bring it up. And then, don't dwell on it. Yes, you're happy about it and you can share the joy. Just don't overdo it. One of Erin's closest friends struggled with infertility. "When I learned I was expecting," Erin said, "I asked her how she'd like me to include her in this season of my life. I said, 'I know this is difficult for you, and I don't want to cause you pain. But you're my friend, and I want to share my excitement if you want me to. How can I be sensitive to you?' Her answer surprised me: 'Just act normal!' was her advice. She had been caused greater pain by pregnant friends who didn't know how to act around her, and so they let the friendship languish and cut her out of their circle. Instead, she wanted to share my excitement and was genuinely happy for me. She was also honest about her feelings: 'The day you told me you were expecting, I went home and cried.' I was glad I asked! I believe we have a stronger friendship as a result."

the baby." Despite the challenges and changes you, your body, and your mate will encounter, here is your guide to finishing what you started—and having fun too!

Month 1

Out of the clear blue, your Clear Blue Easy test showed two lines, or no lines, or a smiley face. Anyway, it displayed beyond a shadow of a doubt that you and the hunka burnin' love are going to be someone's PARENTS. Even if you are delirious with joy about the news, both of you are wearing a deer-in-the headlights look. Yup, this is life-changing stuff, and no one can blame you for not being your regularly amorous self. Wait for the shock to wear off, and maybe your libido will perk up a little. Your mate may immediately notice that your breasts have enlarged (something mine picked up on before I did—go figure), and this may be a rather motivating factor in the whole sex thing. You, my dear, are probably too busy going to the loo every five minutes to consider what was once a pleasant pastime.

Month 2

Since the shock has not really worn off (for you, anyway; he is back to his old randy self) and you have new and alarming symptoms to cope with, sex is probably still not what it was. At this point, you are so fatigued that suddenly you understand how the cat can spend three-quarters of its life snoozing. All you want is a nap—during the day. If you're working, you want to hit the sack at, oh, around 6:30, having ideally been served dinner in bed. Your guy is probably pondering the mysteries of the universe, chief of which is when—if ever—his former lover will again look at him with that twinkle in her eye. Tell him to hold that thought: Your pals tell you that the second trimester is as good as it gets.

Month 3

Last month you probably started feeling nauseated at the slightest provocation. (I didn't want to overwhelm you with that on top of the fatigue.)

And now you are in the throes of the worst feeling of seasickness you've ever encountered, and you're nowhere near a boat. Though Loverboy is still riding high on his great accomplishment of "shooting one past the goalie," or whatever sports metaphor suits his tastes, he is really wondering, "Will we ever hit the sheets again?" Give him a kiss and tell him that the second trimester is right around the corner (although to you the whole idea is about as appealing right now as falling out of an airplane). Then excuse yourself to go throw up.

Month 4

Now we're talkin'. The nausea is waning, and you have more energy than you've had in months. And the idea of sex is starting to sound better and better. After all, it's been, like, three months, as your mate is quick to remind you. Too quick. "What's the matter with you?" you wail. "Isn't the fact that I am carrying YOUR child enough for you? I am growing a HUMAN BEING, and you didn't even get me a CARD for SWEETEST DAY! Is that all you think about—sex, sex, sex?" The hormonal fluctuations are making you feel slightly insane, and the odd look on his face isn't helping.

Month 5

Good news: This may be the best pregnant sex month of all. The hormones swirling in your body, making you morph from the Tooth Fairy to the Wicked Witch of the West on a dime, are also working magic on your libido. Block out the entire month for the likely eventuality that you are going to be interested again—maybe more interested than ever before.

Month 6

You're still in the mood—and how! But your waistline is what they quaintly refer to as "expanding." You feel a bit Buddha-like, and you've begun to wear that oh-so-matronly maternity underwear. How can hubby, still trim and wearing the same briefs or boxers as always, possibly find you, the Incredible Growing Woman, attractive and appealing? Relax. I have it

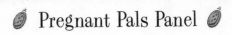

"What Would You Do Differently Next Time?"

"I always hear new moms talk about the 'I wish I'd knowns' of being pregnant and having babies for the first time. I'm curious to know what other first-time mothers wish they had known about pregnancy, so I can learn from their hindsight. If they were pregnant all over again, what would they do differently?"

—WISHFUL IN WISCONSIN

"I would wear a bra every night because it's supposed to help support 'the girls' during that process of going from the Dolly Parton Syndrome to Sucked-Out Shrinkage."

—SARA, 33

"I would take time to meditate, relax, and ponder in my heart the days of my pregnancy. Looking back now, I see how quickly the time went. I was so busy that I didn't take the time to just relax and enjoy being pregnant."

—ANN, 38

"I would complain less about the twenty extra pounds I was lugging around, my backache, and so on, and just enjoy being pregnant."

—TONYA, 26

"I don't think I would have busted my back to keep going to school. I already had one little one at home, and being pregnant, working, and attending the university was too much."

—JULIE, 30

"I would flaunt my belly instead of hating the extra weight."

—JODI, 29

"I wouldn't have played softball at the company picnic when I was eight months pregnant!"

—CHRIS, 28

"I would have skipped the daily trips to the vending machine at work for candy. Those Snickers bars can still be seen on my thighs."

—SUZANNA, 31

"I would have milked it more. Instead of trying to do everything myself, I would have asked for more help. I needed it!"

—SHERRY, 29

"I wouldn't do anything different. My pregnancy was dreamy, special, and perfect. I remember whispering sweet nothings to my growing belly and falling deeper and deeper in love with my daughter even before we met. Pregnancy created the most amazing bond between mother and daughter. We are crazy for each other, even now, seven years later."

—BECKY, 32

on good authority that your man is still raring to go, though he may be worried about hurting the baby. Quote your doctor or *What to Expect* on the fact that sex isn't harmful to Junior and then go "finish the baby."

Month 7

Just between you and me (and *Intended for Pleasure*, of course), things can really heat up as you head into the third inning, so to speak. How can I put this euphemistically? Actually, I can't. But you're a smart girl and you know of what I speak: Between hormones, additional blood flow, and very interesting dream sequences involving your husband, let's just say it will be an explosive month.

Month 8

Just as the dry, dull first trimester becomes a distant memory for your darling mate, the roller-coaster ride starts its inevitable coast downward. For one thing, your belly, though beautiful, is, well, in the way. People more savvy about such matters than I am have suggested alternate contortions to work around this, so by all means, consult those folks. I do have four words of inspiration for you: "Where there's a will…"

Month 9

This is a fascinating month in which your doctor, your boss, and any number of well-wishing friends and relatives (not your parents) will suddenly produce a tip involving your sex life. It's very odd, actually, to have people with whom you sang hymns only moments before come up to you and propose this labor-inducing solution: "Having sex brings it on," they say smugly. "It worked for all four of my labors." Apparently sperm contains oxytocin, a substance of some power that is said to hurry up the proceedings. If you are almost due or overdue and feel like Baby needs a kick-start, try it. (Just so you know, after birth, you and the nice middle-aged lady sharing your hymn book will not return to swapping sex tips. It's just a nine-month, culturally condoned, isolated incident. Trust me.)

What to Do This Month

☐ Sign up for childbirth classes, sibling preparation classes, and a hospital or birth-center tour (if these are not already included in your childbirth class.)

☐ Begin to think about what you need for the baby. Check out sales fliers and garage sales for bargains. For instance, if you know you are going to need a crib and a changing table, take advantage of a store's once-a-year baby sale even if you aren't due for several months.

☐ Buy a "Grandma's Brag Book" type of small photo album for both your mom and your mom-in-law to make them feel special and get them even more excited about their impending new roles.

☐ Journal idea: Tell Baby all about the various relatives he or she is going to inherit. Be detailed. Talk about Grandpa Bucklaschuck's days in minor league baseball, how your sister-in-law's pet mouse recently escaped from his cage, and how Baby's big cousin Grace just learned to walk. You think you will remember all this stuff of life later, but you won't. Your child will come to cherish the ways his family is unique.

Dearest Uncooperative Darling,

Hey, cutes! We kind of (really) wanted to know if you are a boy or a girl, so would it have killed you to help us out a little? You are so silly, sweetie. There we were, Daddy and I, at the ultrasound appointment, dying to know if our family would comprise one boy and one girl or two boys. The ultrasound technician slathered my belly with that cold jelly stuff, and then she roamed around with her magic ultrasound wand. It was just amazing to see you for the first time, to see your beating heart and your kidneys and your lungs. She counted twenty digits—ten fingers and ten toes—and measured your little head. We were so proud of you, just for having normal measurements. But then again, I think every healthy, normal baby is a miracle.

Well, after about 45 minutes of enduring you snoozing with your legs firmly crossed, we decided to take action. The technician suggested I go to the bathroom because that is supposed to wake you up. I gave you a little pep talk when we were alone in that bathroom stall. I also kind of gave you a few gentle shoves to jostle you a bit. It must have worked because you did move around a little. You even grabbed your toes for us. I know you tried, little one, but the technician still couldn't make out exactly what gender you are. When pressed, she said in her estimation you were probably a girl. She was "60 to 70 percent sure," which is interesting but doesn't really answer our burning question. So you're being coy, huh? Oh well, what's life without a little mystery? Besides, it doesn't matter. I thought I wanted a girl when I was pregnant with your brother, and I wouldn't trade him for hundred girls. You love whatever you get, that's the truth, and we love you.

Mama

Month Five

Hubby, Hockey, and Hopping on the Treadmill

And then, suddenly, I felt this tiny ripple, a wave. Instantly that image of the tadpole—an image I'd probably pulled from some high school biology textbook—changed to that of a newborn baby. I knew my baby at that moment looked nothing at all like a newborn, but that was what I was pretending was fluttering inside me. A psychedelic little person doing the breaststroke in a lava lamp.

—from the novel *Midwives* by CHRIS BOHJALIAN

Snapshot! Your baby is between 5.6 and 6.4 inches long and weighs nine ounces. Incredible! She's actually the size of a large banana. Her eyebrows and eyelids are fully developed, and fingernails cover her fingertips. She has begun to make her presence known with little kicks, thrusts, and tossings from side to side. She may be practicing to breathe, and she may even be sucking her itty-bitty thumb.

Watch what you say from here on in. If you talk, read, or sing to your baby, she'll probably be able to hear you. You may want to try reading to her. Either choose some children's classics or read aloud one of your own books. Some studies suggest that a newborn will suck more vigorously when you feed her if you read to her from a book that she frequently heard in utero.

The Birth of a Daddy

When I was pregnant with Ezra, I bought Doyle a gift from the bookstore: *How to Pamper Your Pregnant Wife* by Ron Shultz and Sam Shultz. Of course, he was thrilled, touched to his very core that I would be so thoughtful. Your husband will be too, I'm sure. Be smart, though, and rush out to buy this gem the moment your pregnancy test is positive. Don't wait until the eighth month of your second pregnancy to discover the wealth of wisdom in its pages. Be sure to buy a fat yellow highlighter as a bonus gift so your guy can make the very most of this present. And a couple of new fishing lures and a copy of *Field & Stream* might make the whole package more appealing. After all, the recipient is a guy, and, despite our best efforts, guys have never been known to read pregnancy books.

Men and pregnancy: It can be a strange combination. Someone once said dads-to-be are like immigrants who have one foot in the Old World and one foot in the New. Your husband has a huge stake in your pregnancy, no doubt about it, and the life changes wrought by your growing fetus will affect him as much as you, especially after D-Day, when both of you are faced with protecting, nurturing, and raising an actual child. But for many reasons, pregnancy is *not* the same for men. For one thing, fathers face a challenge in "connecting" with the full experience because they're not the ones feeling queasy, losing their keys every five minutes, or discovering that they're no longer able to zip up their pants (although these points may be debatable—see His Raging Hormones, coming right up).

Writer Keith Bellows discussed this one-foot-in, one-foot-out thing in an article for BabyCenter.com: "Pregnancy is seen as mostly a mom thing. Few women believe that Dad really gets it. And the fact is, we mostly don't. We talk about it. We show interest. We empathize (without going overboard). We even try to read about it, at least a little. But let's face it, our experience of having a baby is virtual and fairly removed until we're face to face with diapering and sleep deprivation. No dad can possibly relate to the minute-by-minute, close-to-the-heart, kick-in-the-gut reality of carrying a baby to term."[1]

Believe it or not though, your mate's mind is probably working overtime trying to adjust to impending fatherhood. He may or may not tell you what's going on inside his head, but male writers, psychologists, and past or presently pregnant dads concur: The father-to-be is definitely chewing on copious quantities of food for thought.

Read of the Month

Now that Baby can hear you loud and clear, start the habit of a bedtime story with *Oh, Baby, the Places You'll Go! A Book to be Read in Utero*, adapted by Tish Rabe from the works of Dr. Seuss. You might feel goofy at first, but I promise this a fun and sweet way to bond with the babe.

Early on in their wives' pregnancies, many men report feeling fear. Armin A. Brott, coauthor with Jennifer Ash of *The Expectant Father*, recalls: "On the one hand, I was still so elated I could barely contain myself; I had visions of walking with my child on the beach, playing, reading, and helping him or her with homework, and I wanted to stop strangers on the street and tell them I was going to be a father. On the other hand, I made a conscious effort to stifle my fantasies and to keep myself from getting attached to the idea of being pregnant. That way, if we had a miscarriage or something else went wrong, I wouldn't be devastated."[2]

Your mate may also be dealing with other kinds of worries. Will he be a good father? Will his job be good enough to provide for a growing family, especially if he is now to be the sole breadwinner? Will his relationship with you ever be the same?

Jerrold Shapiro, Ph.D., author of *When Men Are Pregnant*, adds that a surprising number of men actually fret about how they will react in the delivery room. "More than 80 percent of the fathers I come across in my practice say they were worried they wouldn't be able to [carry out their duties] when their wife was in labor," he writes. "They were afraid of passing out, throwing up, or getting queasy in the presence of all those bodily fluids. Such fears may be based on cartoons and sitcoms and our culture's way of making fun of men, but two things became clear: The men all expected it—and it almost never happens. In follow-up interviews, it turned out only one out of six hundred men fainted, and that was in August in Fresno [California], and the air conditioning had gone out and two of the nurses had to leave the room, too."

Dr. Shapiro has also noticed that men can be afraid of "women's medicine." Unless your husband happens to be a gynecologist, he may be a bit apprehensive about the ob-gyn planet. "Even as observers, many men feel dehumanized, embarrassed, and inhibited around stirrups and gynecological exams," he writes. "Hospital examining rooms and delivery rooms are not made comfortable for a father. Men are usually fairly ignorant about

 His Raging Hormones?!

"Expectant moms aren't the only ones going through big changes. According to a new Canadian study, dads-to-be also experience hormonal fluctuations during their partners' pregnancies. Researchers tested blood samples from thirty-four couples in prenatal classes. 'We found that the men's levels of prolactin and cortisol increased and decreased in patterns similar to those of their pregnant partner,' says Anne Storey, Ph.D., a professor of psychology at Memorial University of Newfoundland in St. Johns. 'Though their symptoms were less dramatic, the fathers also showed changes in appetite, fatigue, irritability, and weight gain.' These same hormones may play a role in making men more nurturing toward their babies."[3]

—*Parents Expecting*, Winter 2000-2001

a woman's reproductive system—it's what happens 'down there.' And so when men encounter all this for the first time, they get clobbered with it."[4]

How to Be a Supportive Pregnant Wife

Despite all the fears swirling around in their new-daddy heads, most guys truly want to participate in their wife's pregnancies. There are definite ways you can make this easier—or harder—for your guy. After all, you have certain expectations of how he should be acting and how he should be treating you. And those expectations may or may not have anything to do with reality.

Case in point: Growing up, I saw my dad treat my mom to something special on the twelfth of every month. He would give her a card, some flowers, or some other little thing to commemorate their wedding anniversary, which fell on September 12. Consequently, I came to my own marriage expecting Doyle to bear tokens of affection for me on the ninth of every month. Was I in for a rude awakening? Definitely. There have been no "monthaversary" celebrations for us since our first month of dating. But really, I have to admit this particular expectation was somewhat unfair. Doyle is a wonderful husband, and without hesitation I'd take his stellar qualities over a Hallmark card and a carnation any month. All that to say, watch your expectations. Pay attention to them.

And don't compare husbands either, unless you're making a favorable comparison (in which case keep it to yourself around girlfriends whose husbands are complete thugs.) My friend Heather has this amazing mate who seems to cater to her every whim. I've seen him follow her around the house and ask her if she needs a back rub. I personally wish he would give how-to-be-a-great-husband seminars, but he's too busy grinding cloves for his homemade aromatherapy massage oil.

I'm guessing that your husband—like mine—falls somewhere between Love Slave and Knuckle-Dragging Caveman. You know your man better than anyone, and you know how he shows his love. There's no point in comparing him to the Back-Rub Boys out there, bless all five of them. Remember that your husband is probably freaking out a bit too. After all, his world is about to change drastically. Here are a few ways to ease your guy's mind and facilitate his greater participation in your fabulous "joint project."

Acknowledge his feelings. Initiate conversation about some of the fears and concerns he may have. And don't laugh at them. As it is, your hormones and the resulting lunacy will give him plenty of reason to laugh at *you.*

Celebrate his role. You will make him feel much more a part of your pregnancy if you meaningfully and intentionally call attention to his new role. Search for ways to involve him in these nine months of expectation. One neat idea is to visit BabyCenter.com and sign him up for a weekly e-mail update on your pregnancy. Getting a weekly e-mail at work or at home with a description and a picture of how his baby is growing and changing will surely fascinate him.

Be your guy's clipping service. Celebrities and corporations hire clipping services to search out any print media that pertains to them. Since your husband probably won't read *What to Expect When You're Expecting* cover to cover, you can highlight the main points for him. The same goes for magazine articles. You're reading like a fiend anyway; you may as well pick out some material you think he might be interested in. I have found that a "Hey, when you get a chance, here's this interesting article on sex and pregnancy [just to name a topic of interest]—it's really funny and well-written" works much better than "You never read any of my pregnancy books. You don't even care about me or this baby!"

Consult him on everything (within reason). Don't assume that just because you're a woman you know infinitely more than he ever will on the topic of pregnancy and babies. If you want him to be involved, ask him his opinion on everything: prenatal tests, pesticides, nursery themes, names, whether you will work or not after the baby comes, whether you should have a home birth or deliver at the hospital, and so on. In short, involve him whenever you can in every aspect of your experience.

Don't ask leading questions. I know I am guilty of this, as most pregnant women are, but it's hard on a guy when his wife constantly harangues him about her weight gain. My former boss was always exasperated with his wife, who would ask him, "Do you think I am too fat?" "There is absolutely no right answer for that question!" he pointed out. "I mean, you can't say yes—no two ways about that—but what can you say? 'No, dear, you're just fat enough'?" (I know of one guy, a total meathead who shall remain nameless, who would tease his pregnant wife about her size and say things in birthing class like "Roll over, big girl." *Big girl?* Well, enough said.) If you're feeling insecure about your growing girth, consider just saying so. But not too often. I imagine any guy would prefer his wife simply asking him to please tell her once in a while that he still thinks she's beautiful rather than be faced with endless backhanded, whiny questions for which no satisfactory answer exists.

Hey, girls, now that I've covered some ways you can be a better pregnant wife, let's turn the tables and shoot some strategies out there for the guy-folk. After all, you're the one who's pregnant. Your man needs to know how he can be the best possible support for you through all of this, and, having never been p.g. himself, he may be somewhat clueless about how to proceed. So here's what I'm thinking: Even though I know this is a colossal generalization, and you may even be insulted by it, I've decided to use a sports metaphor to describe winning and losing ways of being a daddy-to-be. In your household, you could very well be the one clutching the remote during Monday night football while your hubby curls up in a chair to read a novel. It happens.

Just for fun, though, and because I happen to be slightly obsessed with the sport myself, I've decided to play around with some hockey terms to get my point across. You know—to use his "love language." (My husband has astutely pointed out that this is also *my* own love language, but I digress.) So dog-ear the page or stick a bookmark right here and pass the book over to your main man. This month's Nifty Nine tips belong to him.

(If right now he's watching the Super Bowl, or the Final Four, or the World Series, you may want to wait until halftime or another appropriate moment. If in fact he is watching Hockey Night in Canada, his beloved team is in the hunt for the Stanley Cup, and the game is in triple overtime, now is not the time to shove a book under his nose. Now is also not the time to suggest food, drink, or even the act of marital love between two consenting adults. The thing is, he's not in a consenting frame of mind. He's in a hockey-crazed coma.)

Make Yourself a Hall of Fame Dad-to-Be: The Nifty Nine Power Plays for Pregnant Pops

This is a section especially for my male readers (hi, Dad!) and for the mates of my female ones. Let's talk hockey for a minute. You may be more of a soccer guy or a football freak like my own dear husband, but hockey is my sport, and surely you've read enough *Sports Illustrated* or *ESPN: The Magazine* to have a grasp on the basics.

What follows is a bit of coaching on how to really be there for your pregnant wife, to stand above the underperformers out there who really should be sent to the minors for marital mediocrity. After all, she's your wife—the love of your life—and she is carrying your child/offspring/progeny/heir apparent. No one expects you to blubber like a baby over Paul Anka's tune "Having My Baby" or to wear one of those fake pregnancy prostheses all the time (or at least not to the office). But listen up: With all the hormonal nuttiness and physical changes going on in your wife's body, she is playing short-handed, so to speak. This is where you get to come in, sharp in the slot, aggressive along the boards, and always, always alert to scoring a goal. *Whaddya mean "scoring a goal"?* you might be thinking. *I already one-timed it in from the blue line. What more do you want?* I want to see you hustle out there and produce like crazy! Your wife needs you, Junior needs you, and the team needs you in order to play at full strength.

1. Serve and Protect

It may not seem like much, and it's not, to be frank, but you will need to take over any duties that involve substances harmful to the baby. Because prolonged exposure to weed killer, insecticide, fertilizer, and so on has been linked to birth defects, you will have to take over the gardening and lawn jobs. Not so bad, huh? Maybe you already do that. Well, before you get too excited, you are now compelled to clean the cat litter, too, even if it's her cat and your secret nickname for it is "Roadkill." Cat feces are chock-full of the parasite found in raw meats—not at all good for Junior.

2. Go, Hunter-Gatherer, and Hunt Down the Food at Piggly Wiggly and Bring It to a Place Where She Can Find It

Early in the pregnancy, your wife may get queasy from the food smells at the grocery store. And by the third trimester, lugging big bags of food around is a bad, not to mention painful, proposition.

3. Keep an Eye on Baby

Have you ever heard the saying that a tied game is like "kissing your sister"? Hearing about your baby's milestones secondhand is just the same. Sure, it's nice and all, but it definitely lacks the power and grandeur of the big, emotional win. So go to as many doctor's appointments as you can. Your gal needs you there for the ultrasound at the very least. The second most important appointment will be when you hear Baby's first heartbeat. (And unquestionably, if there should be any special tests, such as an amniocentesis, do not let her go it alone.) Attending these will help you feel more like an involved, invested coach than a fan up in the nosebleed section.

4. Take Your Wacko Wife in Stride

So what if she snapped at you for wearing navy socks with black pants? (Okay, so she *cried* about it.) Ron Shultz, in his groundbreaking work *How to Pamper Your Pregnant Wife*, describes what may be going on in your usually happy home: "One nanosecond, your wife may be totally content with herself and you, her loving husband. Then, *whammo!* Before the fall of the next nanosecond, she's suddenly berating you for being totally inconsiderate because you wouldn't eat the strawberry pie her mother baked for you six months earlier—even though strawberries make you break out into a rash."[5] These times may be trying, as my husband can attest to, but remember, those agitated hormones are hip-checking your wife into the boards of life—hard. Take it from Wayne Gretzky. When asked how he had coped with his pregnant wife's mood swings, he responded in a true Hall of Fame manner: "Pregnancy's tough at times for any woman. You've got to be there when it's tough for your wife. That's what husbands are for."[6] No wonder they call him the Great One.

5. Don't Ever, Under Any Circumstances, Say, "Boy, You Sure Are Getting Big"

Strike words such as "large," "rotund," and especially "chubby" from your vocabulary immediately. Even if in your mind "big" means "blossoming," and you are referring solely to her growing belly, she takes it to mean "fat." This is a touchy subject, my friends. Even if she badgers you within an inch of your life, never, *never* comment on her weight gain except to say she looks beautiful to you. Also, don't comment on her eating habits. If the woman wants to eat seven cream-filled donuts for breakfast, just sit there like a mute and pass the napkins. Any infractions of the above guidelines will result in a penalty, at the very least Two Minutes for Insensitivity, if not Game Misconduct.

6. Go with the Nesting Urge

At some point during the pregnancy, your mate will no doubt be seized with the urge to nest. You're probably thinking it's a bunch of garbage; I thought so too until I felt compelled to rearrange my pajama drawer according to color. Don't put off her urgent wishes for you to assemble the crib. Do it. She absolutely has to have things in order, and if that means you find yourself installing the car seat three months before the due date, just roll with it.

7. Be Your Wife's Health Partner

You know that exercise will benefit your wife like crazy. It will give her stamina now and strength for labor. And you know that whole grains and fresh fruits and vegetables are the best nourishment for her and Junior. Also, caffeine should be limited to a cup or so a day. All that to say that your efforts to encourage her (which does not mean "badger her") to build healthy habits will go a long way. Forming good habits and breaking bad ones is always easier when you have a buddy, so work out with her, pass up the hot dog for a turkey sandwich on whole grain, and switch to half-and-half coffee. Who knows? You may both get into great shape!

8. Get in the Game

Brag. Rave. Enthuse. Getting into your wife's pregnancy and the whole idea of becoming a father will mean the world to her. Check out web sites about pregnancy, read baby-name books with her, and compare consumer reports on car seats. If you sign up for a birthing class, be there with bells on. You're in this thing together, and she needs to know you're in the game 100 percent.

9. Pamper Your Wife

Do some absolutely sweet, totally unexpected thing to spoil your lady. Take her shopping for maternity clothes (propose this while she's sitting down), learn to give a great back rub (or at least give her a gift certificate for a massage), fix her breakfast in bed, spring for flowers. Guys, this is truly Hall of Fame material here. I'm talking Guy LaFleur, Marcel Dionne, Gordie Howe. So go above and beyond the call of duty and do some thoughtful, extraordinary things for her over the next few months. She will think you are a superstar.

Exercise? Have You Completely Lost Your Mind?

I know what you're thinking: *You expect me, great with child, to burn calories?* I know, I know. Working out during pregnancy, especially during the first and last trimesters, is about as appealing as bunion surgery. I worked out during my first pregnancy. Once. On the treadmill. For ten minutes. At the time, I thought that was quite enough, thank you very much. My second time around, though, I actually put the pedal to the metal and made myself exercise at least twice a week during the entire nine months.

You know it by now: I won't lie to you. Though supposedly in some semblance of a fit state, my bod is still less than fabulous. No one would confuse my post-pregnant form with that of—say—Cindy Crawford's. I even gained more weight the second time. A lot more. My husband tried to comfort me with the ol' "muscle weighs more than fat" shtick. Of course, he's right, but surely my semiburly *latissimus dorsi* couldn't account for my new ten pounds. I tried to keep two things in mind: Every pregnancy is different, and trying to trim back weight gain is really one of the last things to be worried about. Having said that, I can now turn my attention to you, my pregnant reader, who may be utterly revolted by the thought of exercising.

You gotta try it, girlfriend. *But, but, but, but, but—isn't there some kind of set-in-concrete rule about not starting an exercise program while pregnant if you weren't previously in one?* Nope. Don't shoot me—I'm just the messenger—but that old wives' tale went the way of leg warmers and Jordache jeans. *But it's a known fact that you shouldn't overdo it during pregnancy. Doesn't this mean "no exercise"?* Not exactly. Sorry to dash your visions of popping bonbons day after blissfully pampered day, but you can do yourself a heap of favors by incorporating some kind of fitness regime into your pregnant life. (But do be sure to talk to your doctor before starting any exercise program.) Yes, it is easier to exercise through pregnancy if you were in the habit beforehand, but even if the most strenuous exercise you've done in the last six years has been carrying grocery bags to your car, you can start getting more fit any time. That's not to say, of course, that one can go from sofa sluggard to Boston Marathon hopeful during pregnancy. You've got to tailor any kind of exercise to your existing condition *and* to your physician's recommendations.

Carol Stahmann Dilfer, author of *Your Baby, Your Body: Fitness During Pregnancy*, provides a solid answer to the "why bother?" question: "A weak, flabby, deconditioned body can deliver a baby—no doubt about it—but it pays for it later [with] aching shoulders, tight inner thighs, sore perineal area, fatigue. Oh! The fatigue," she writes. "A strong conditioned body, on the other hand, fares much better. It may labor as long as the flabby body, but it will work much more easily and efficiently. And it will not be nearly as fatigued by the work."

The demands of labor aside, you won't believe the bonuses of a fit, strong, pregnant bod. Work with me, girls, and I promise you'll thank me later.

Boost your energy! Pregnancy can make you feel blah, but regular exercise will make you feel as if you can at least get through the day with a little more pep. Exercise also invigorates your cardiovascular system, so you don't poop out so fast. Plus, strong, toned muscles means it takes less effort to do absolutely anything, be it fixing dinner or decorating the nursery.

Build stamina for labor! "It makes perfect sense," Dilfer says. "The better shape you're in, the stronger you'll be come labor and delivery time. Giving birth is akin to running a marathon—it requires stamina, determination, and focus. Training for childbirth through exercise ensures success."[7]

Banish discomfort! Exercise lengthens and strengthens your muscles, which helps you sit and stand straighter, reducing the aches and pains of pregnancy. Stretches relieve back pain, walking improves your circulation, and swimming tones your abdominal muscles.

Sleep tight! Many women complain of pregnancy insomnia, a condition surely aggravated in later months by efforts to find a comfy position. Working out tuckers you out enough so you'll fall asleep faster. Exercise may even make for a slumber so deep you won't wake up to roll over or visit the bathroom.

Reduce stress and lift your spirits! Have I mentioned hormones? Those rambunctious forces may have you feeling fretful, stressed, and/or blue. Exercise ups your levels of serotonin, a brain chemical linked to mood, putting you in a better frame of mind for finessing all the ups and downs.

Improve your self-image! Okay, so your weight is at a lifetime high these days, and you can't bump into someone at the mall without, well, bumping into them. Exercise can truly help you feel better about your body. Even though you feel a bit like a moose with a beer gut some days, it will help a little to remember that your bicep is nice and toned. Not that anyone will notice, but you'll know. Bonus: I promise you that any exercise you do will win you the admiration of friends, family, and strangers alike. Warning: You may get looks at the gym, especially from single guys. Well, not those kinds of looks from single guys, believe me. What I mean is alarmed looks, ones that say, "Whoa! She's gonna have a baby right here, right now!" Other than that particular demographic, the population at large will think you're a hero.

Bounce back after birth! This is one benefit that should loom large as you contemplate whether to lace up your running shoes or slide on your bunny slippers: Exercise means you'll get your old body back faster. I'm not promising you'll zip up your pre-baby jeans at the hospital. (If you do, don't tell anyone, least of all a fellow female. No one but you and your husband will find this to be charming in the least. Plus, I just don't want to know.) When you've worked at keeping up your strength and muscle tone all through your pregnancy, your body will have an easier time bouncing back after you give birth.

Great Exercises for Great Pregnant Bods

Walking. Incredibly easy, cheap, and accessible, walking will keep you fit without jarring your knees and ankles. A lot of women, though, use the walking option as a cop out. They will walk, but not at the intensity required for a decent workout. Don't be one of them. Instead, work it as you walk.

Swimming. Swimming is the perfect pregnancy workout. When you swim you work large muscle groups (arms and legs), tone your butt and abs, get some cardio benefits, and the list goes on. Check out *Fit Pregnancy* magazine for aquacise ideas or join an aqua-aerobics class at a local gym or health club. The best part is how amazing you will feel—buoyant, loose, and free—despite the extra pounds you are lugging around. So throw on your cute maternity suit and jump in.

Flexibility and strength training. Stretching, when done properly, is a balm to aching limbs, can give you long and lean muscles, and keep you limber with little if any impact on your joints.

Kegels. According to a BabyCenter.com poll, 41 percent of pregnant women did their Kegels once in a while, 34 percent several times a day, 10 percent once a day, and 15 percent performed these little exercises a few times a week. You should shoot for three or four sets of ten Kegels, three times a day. Why? These easy, do-them-anywhere-anytime exercises have numerous benefits, chief of which is retaining your ability to convulse with giggles and/or sneeze without having a little "gee, wasn't my face *red*" accident. They also reduce hemorrhoids, strengthen the walls of your vagina, and—*bonus!*—give you better orgasms. (As Martha would say, "That's a good thing.")

Weight training. If you get expert guidance, learn good techniques, and take the necessary precautions, weight training will be a great way to tone and strengthen your muscles. And you won't believe the difference it makes. "Women often underestimate the amount of upper body strength they will need for pregnancy and afterward," writer Dana Sullivan told *Fit*

Exercise and You: An Interview with Personal Trainer and Pregnant Pal Kristi Tuck

Q: Is it true that if you didn't work out before pregnancy, you shouldn't start a workout program now?

A: Absolutely not. That is really a big myth for some reason. I think a lot of women use that as an excuse to not exercise, but the truth is, you can start an exercise program at any point during your pregnancy if you haven't had complications.

It's possible to have a very low level of fitness before you become pregnant, then start a good program, and end up far more fit during and after your pregnancy than you were before. This is because, pregnant or not, your body responds to strength training the same way: If you fatigue a muscle, it will become stronger. The key is to check your exercise plans out with your doctor first and to do everything in moderation. Any form of exercise done gradually and safely is great. If you didn't have a routine of high-impact workouts (spinning, step aerobics, and body pump classes) before, you shouldn't start now.

Q: What special considerations should pregnant women keep in mind as they work out?

A: The biggest concern is overheating. If your body gets too hot, you will draw blood away from your core—the baby—to your muscles, which are working overtime. So pay attention to your body. If you feel as if you can't carry on a conversation, you are overdoing it. Also, your muscles are going to fatigue faster, so adapt your workout and don't lift more than feels comfortable. After sixteen weeks, don't lie on your back for sit ups or weight training. The added weight of your uterus puts pressure on the veins to the heart and the blood supply to the baby.

Q: What kinds of exercises are best for pregnancy?

A: The pool is the best thing of all. [Aquatic exercise] will help reduce swelling and is nonimpact. But unless you are a serious swimmer, you may not know how to get your heart rate up high enough, so you may just dilly-dally around. Still, time in the pool will make your back and muscles feel better anyway. Also, any kind of stretching exercise really helps as far as maintaining a correct posture. Certain kinds of abdominal [exercises] are really great for pregnant women. A lot of people think you can't work your abs when you are expecting, but the opposite is true. Just don't do sit-ups after the fourth month. Join a "Maternity in Motion" class at a gym or buy a pregnancy workout video. Kathy Kaehler and Kathi Smith have both developed sensible and effective workouts (for pregnancy) that are excellent. Finally, moderate weight training is wonderful because you can really use that muscular endurance for pushing during labor.

Q: How soon can I work out after I deliver?

A: It all depends on your delivery. For a vaginal birth, you can begin working out four weeks after you give birth. For a C-section, you should wait six weeks, even eight. As long as you're not cramping and bleeding and you feel good, you can start working out. Listen to your body. It will tell you if you are overdoing it. Even a few days after delivering, you can start with the toning exercises. Do your Kegels, leg lifts—those kinds of things. You will bounce back faster after birth if you've been working out. No matter what level of fitness you pursue during your pregnancy, exercise during those months makes a huge difference postpartum.

Kristi Tuck is fitness director at the Michigan Athletic Club. Her daughter, Emma, is four months old.

Pregnancy magazine. During pregnancy, strong back and shoulder muscles make it easier to stand up straight. And after? "You'll be amazed at how often you need upper body strength just to get through the day," she adds.[8] It's true. Between hauling the baby-carrier-car-seat-thing around and lugging loads of laundry, you'll be a chiropractic nightmare-in-waiting without toned back muscles. Weights also build bone strength, which is especially important during pregnancy when women are at a higher risk of losing bone density.

 ## Thank You, Arnold!

Here's a tip for when you make it to the hot seat on *Who Wants to Be a Millionaire?* Kegels are named after Dr. Arnold Kegel, a gynecologist who advocated them in the 1940s to help his post-partum patients check incontinence.

Fitness-for-two classes. If you're anything like me, actually participating in a group exercise class is about as appealing as that trig final from high school that still gives you nightmares. While pregnant with Ezra, I did hook up with a class specifically designed for pregnant women, and it proved to be better than I thought. For one thing, everyone was in the same rare form and experiencing similar types of things such as sciatic nerve troubles, baby-naming dilemmas, maternity clothing woes, and the like. From that point of view, classes provide an excellent way to bond with some new pregnant pals. (Of course, not everyone could share my feeling-like-a-tugboat issues. There was one woman, Paloma, who looked as if she had pranced right off the pages of Italian *Vogue*. She had long, lean limbs and this nominal bulge sticking straight out of her center, a bulge most people would think was cute. None of this innertube-around-the-middle business for Paloma. Anyway, I'm sure she was a very nice woman, but I still had to pray for grace when I noticed that she was wearing a thong leotard. Did I mention she was about 8 months pregnant at this juncture? My own underwear situation was far more practical, I consoled myself, as I considered the Grandma Walton Big Coverage Specials I wore under my sweats.) Italian supermodels aside, these classes really are great. Not only will you have the assurance of knowing every move you make is safe and beneficial for baby, but you'll also be motivated by peer pressure to keep going even when you'd rather be at the juice bar nursing a banana smoothie.

He or She?

Will it be snails and puppy dog tails or sugar and spice? Inquiring minds—the grocery store clerk, the in-laws, the neighbors, and definitely you—want to know. Even though you would probably state for the record that all you want is a healthy baby, which in and of itself is quite true, the question of gender probably consumes you for at least part of the day, every day.

I was sure beyond a doubt that Jonah was a girl. In fact, everyone was sure. Out of my collection of girlfriends, all but two felt positive I would have a girl. "I can't picture you with anything but a girl—you're so girlie," one of them explained. That seemed to be the general consensus. I couldn't even imagine myself with a boy. I would daydream about decorating the nursery with a great girls' literature theme, and I scoured used bookstores for well-preserved copies of *Anne of Green Gables, Rebecca of Sunnybrook Farm,* and *Little House on the Prairie.* We already had three wonderful, rough-and-tumble nephews on Doyle's side. (These were our "practice" children, courtesy of Doyle's sister Jodi.) A girl was due, so surely we were a shoo-in for the X chromosome.

So when the ultrasound technician pronounced, beyond the shadow of a reasonable doubt, that our baby was a boy (she even gave us a photo of his penis to show off to the public), we were stunned. I admit I felt a

"I'm So Disappointed We're Not Having a Girl!"

I just I had my amnio, and I found out I'm having a boy. I'm shocked, as I was sure it was a girl, and I don't want to admit it, but I am so disappointed. I feel guilty and horrible, but I really wanted a girl. Of course my husband is ecstatic, so I haven't been able to talk to him about it. How can I feel better?

—DREAMING OF A DAUGHTER IN DELAWARE

Dear Dreaming,

I was pregnant with my third child in three years. My first two were boys. I wanted a little girl. I saw pink and lace and fluff everywhere I went. My husband and I decided this would be our last child, and we took permanent measures to ensure that it would be. Then came the sonogram—and with it, the image of a little something extra on my "daughter." My hopes were shattered.

Now I should point out that I had had some spotting in the beginning of this pregnancy. I should have been overjoyed that the baby was healthy and that the pregnancy was progressing beautifully. But those weren't my main thoughts. I was sad. On the way home I cried. I felt so guilty about being sad, but the guilt didn't take away the weight on my heart. I decided to give myself time to grieve the daughter I would never have. I grieved the fact that I wouldn't have a little girl who looked just like me. No pink dresses. No girls' nights out. No passing on the skills to my daughter that my mom had taught me and her mom had taught her.

Amazingly, once I gave myself permission to be sad, it didn't take too long before I was okay with having three sons. My boys (now 10, 8, and 7) are best friends. They love each other. That third son that I struggled with in the beginning, Ryan, is the one who tells me that I'm the best mom and that I make the best homemade pizza. His favorite question to ask is "Mom, can I love you forever?" Then he gives me a great big hug and kiss. He is my lover. Every mom needs a child like Ryan.

But my story doesn't end there. I began praying that the Lord would show me what to do with this desire to have a daughter. Should I somehow become involved with little girls? I could teach a Sunday school class. I could become a Big Sister. Perhaps I could volunteer as a Girl Scout leader. The Lord led my husband and me down the road of adoption. Four years later, when a young girl asked us to adopt her baby (four sonograms clearly showed it to be a girl), we were ready! I would not exchange any of my children for another. If Ryan had been a girl, we never would have known the blessing of Amanda, and that would truly have been a tragedy. You can't always see right away the magnitude of blessings God plans to give you.

So give yourself some time to be sad. It's okay. But then move on to the great gift God has bestowed upon you. Chances are, that baby you thought should have been a girl (or boy) is exactly what you need.

—JODI CONNELL, 31, MOTHER OF MICHAEL, 11, JACOB, 10, RYAN, 8, AND AMANDA, 4 pang of disappointment. Visions of darling Easter dresses, quaint tea parties, and mother-daughter trips to Prince Edward Island, site of the Anne stories, flew out the window.

But almost immediately those fond hopes for a daughter were replaced by a crackle of excitement. A boy. A boy! Our son. We loved this baby already, so he certainly had that going for him. Suddenly new visions danced in my mind: I would teach the little guy to skate and to love

 Fun and Frivolous Gender Predictors

In her whimsical, clever little book, *Boy or Girl: 50 Fun Ways to Find Out,* Shelly Lavigne offers fifty flippant tests, collected from folk wisdom from around the world, to help you guess your baby's sex. Here are a few of her tests you can try at home, alone or with your main man, or at a baby shower with a gaggle of giggly pals:

- Stare into the mirror for at least one minute, but not more than three. Do your eyes dilate? Boy oh boy. They don't? You're having a girl.

- After seven months, check out your waistline, or lack thereof. If your belly is straight up and down, you're in for lots of quality time with dump trucks and steam shovels. But, Lavigne says, "bulging sides go along with a girl." (Girls are also said to be heralded by more significant weight gain, fatter legs, and a bigger backside.)

- Here's one for those of you whose favorite subject was chemistry: Add one tablespoon of crystal Drano to your first-of-the-morning urine and wait a bit to see what happens. Bluish-Yellow = Boy; Greenish-Brown = Girl.[9]

hockey as much as his mama, Opa, and Uncle Dan did. He would have the bluest of eyes, inherited from his good-looking Pa. I'd dress him in adorable, handsome little denim overalls and plan a mother-son trip to see the polar bears in Churchill, Manitoba. Fishing, hunting, and football flashed through Doyle's mind, and neither of us could wipe the smile off our faces.

When we got home from this momentous ultrasound appointment, a present was waiting for our son. A sportswriter friend had spent the afternoon interviewing hockey legend Gordie Howe, and he had thoughtfully had Mr. Howe autograph a puck for our baby. Our friend had no idea we were going to have a boy, but Someone in a much higher position did. Not to say that a puck isn't a perfectly suitable gift for a baby girl—chicks with sticks are cool—but somehow that round piece of rubber seemed to be a very personal message of affirmation, blessing, and joyful tidings.

You love what you get. I can't repeat that often enough, and you'll know that truth for yourself true when your baby's gender is revealed. About half of you will opt to find out—if you can—at your 20-week ultrasound appointment. The rest of you will want a surprise. Even if you don't want to know, for sure, until they declare it one way or the other in the delivery room, it's fun to speculate madly. (If you don't guess, you can be quite sure that strangers on the street will take a stab at it, judging baby's gender by how high, low, or sideways you are carrying.)

What to Do This Month

☐ Decide where you will have the baby—at home, at which hospital or birthing center, or...? Also, select your birthing coach. Your husband is your best choice, of course, but if for some reason he can't participate, choose your labor coach (perhaps your mom, sister, or best friend) with care.

☐ Start thinking about a birth plan, a strategy for what kind of birthing experience you really want. (See chapter 9 for more on pain-management options.)

☐ Join a fitness class for pregnant women or a water aerobics class. If you can't find a class, find a good exercise video tailored for expectant moms (look back at Exercise and You). For optimum fun, find a pregnant pal to share the misery, er, benefits of regular exercise.

☐ Journal idea: Tell Baby all about her daddy, his likes and dislikes, dreams and aspirations. Include funny stories about him, his unique quirks, and his sterling qualities. Even better, have the main man himself be a guest writer for this section of your journal.

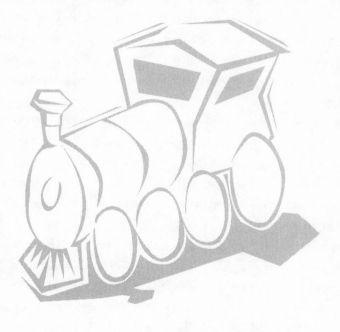

Well then, little one, my Phoebe or my Ezra.

When I was doing research for my baby-name book, *A Is for Adam*, the names *Ezra* and *Phoebe* just jumped out as front-runners. I wanted both my girl's name and my boy's name to be from the Bible, and I wanted names that would match your big brother's—Jonah—in terms of style and originality. *Ezra* is a vibrant Hebrew name. I love that he was a writer, such a wonderful leader, and truly an unsung hero. (Plus I adore the letter Z!) *Phoebe* means "bright shining star." Isn't that gorgeous? I appreciate that it's a classic name, dating back to the ancient Greeks, and it's well used in literature too. But the biggest reason for my attraction? I admire the biblical Phoebe, a deaconess who delivered the book of Romans for Paul and who might have written Hebrews too. (I like to think she did!)

They say that now you can hear me and maybe even your daddy and your big brother Jonah. You can hear our new dog Dinah barking, and they say you can hear the vacuum cleaner. Unfortunately, you won't be able to hear that because it never runs! Although now that Dinah is shedding all over the place, Daddy bought a Dustbuster, and we've been vacuuming more now than in our whole married lives.

So, squirmy, what's up with all the wiggling? Last night you kicked up a storm at the Faith Hill concert, but then when Tim McGraw came out you quieted right down. (They also say unborn babes like yourself prefer classical music, in which case you're in trouble 'cause around here it's all blues and pop and rock.) I seem to feel you most around midnight and then later, once again right before morning comes. Is it my imagination, or are you more wriggly than your brother was? I hope that you are exactly who you are, even though we are putting in our requests for a calm little one who is mellow and likes books! Whoever you are, we love you and can't wait to show you around.

Sweet dreams, baby mine.

Love,
Mama

Duncan/Dylan, Dagmar/Daisy, Ditziness and Dreams

Talk to any parent who has ever named a baby, and you'll see that names are the most distilled love poems. Fashioned from only a few syllables, a name carries a precious cargo of private meanings, memories of revered relationships, rich associations, and only the bravest hopes.
—MIMI READ, *Martha Stewart Baby*

Snapshot! Now we're talking. Your baby is doing tae bo in your belly, and you're really becoming vested in the idea that you're going to be a mommy. Because he is probably lulled to sleep during the day by all your comings and goings, it's party time at night when you're about ready for ten solid hours of shuteye. His eyelids may have parted, and his eyes may be open. It's even possible that he could survive if you went into early labor, but give him a good pep talk and tell him to wait a few more months. He'll be happy he did.

"Untitled Baby Project"

My friends Lisa and Paulo Freire are in the process of naming their baby, who is due in a few months. Let's sneak up on them and eavesdrop on their discussion, one which I'm sure will ring a bell with most of you out there in the throes of "naming fever." Like most couples who are trying to come up with a suitable tag for their offspring, the Freires are not reaching a decision easily. While negotiations aren't going badly, exactly, neither are they progressing smoothly:

"As long as she agrees with me, I don't have a problem," Paulo jokes.

"He likes very, very few names," she says ominously.

"Well, that's okay," Paulo says, "because I plan to have very few kids."

Luckily for Paulo, his wife laughs at this, but she isn't ready to wave the white flag yet.

"You are too picky," she accuses. "For instance, what's wrong with 'Hannah'?"

"I told you. It's the same backward and forward."

"That's a reason not to like a name?" Lisa shakes her head.

Clearly, the naming of Baby Freire is not imminent.

As it is for many parents, the prospect of naming your bundle of joy may be exciting but somewhat daunting. Should you honor a family member by making Baby a namesake? What about choosing a name that pays tribute to your cultural heritage? Is it better to bestow your child with an offbeat, unusual name, or is it kinder to give a name that ensures he or she won't be teased on the playground?

"Naming a baby can literally consume nine months," says Bruce Lansky, author of several baby-name books, including *The Baby Name Survey Book.* "You can argue with your spouse, and it can be a really intense process. It can also be really fun."

My first book, *A Is for Adam: Biblical Baby Names,* is different from most name books, which give a huge, dictionary-like listing of every name from Aab to Zuli. Instead of merely listing every name from the Bible—and there are over 3000—I plucked the most attractive, viable, and meaningful (in my opinion) 125 and profiled each one. As I wrote *Adam,* I assumed that today's parents want a name for their baby that is fresh, beautiful, and stylistically suited to their tastes. But in the process I also learned that they want something more. In my research, I was amazed by how many young parents wanted their offspring's moniker to mean something, to reflect some character quality, their cultural heritage, a spiritual reference, or some slice of family history that is deeply meaningful to them.

B Is for Boaz

I may be biased towards Bible names. (I've written a book about them, and both my children possess handles from Scripture.) The Bible is not only God-breathed revelation, but also a sensational source of names, especially for parents of faith. With more than half of the fifty most popular boys' names hailing from the Bible, it's obvious that baby namers from all creeds are drawn to Scripture. From Adam to Zachary and Abigail to Zorah, the pages of the Good Book are rife with spiritually meaningful namesakes. Where once Nathan and Rebekah were almost certainly someone's Jewish grandparents, now playgrounds are inhabited by cheeky little Noahs and pint-sized Hannahs.

 Read of the Month

Check out the library or your favorite nook for books. It's time to get serious about baby names! My favorite volumes include *Baby Names Now* and *Beyond Jennifer and Jason, Madison and Montana*, both by Pamela Satran and Linda Rosenkrantz; *Puffy, Xena, Uma, and Quentin* by Joal Ryan; and of course, *A Is for Adam* by yours truly.

By giving their babies Bible names, parents may hope that Noah's faith, Lydia's industriousness, Tabitha's kindness, or Caleb's boldness will rub off on their namesakes—or at least inspire them to live up to the best qualities that their names evoke.

Besides turning to the Bible, there are other ways to rise above generic baby naming and choose for your child a moniker rich with meaning. Parents-to-be for whom "so many books, so little time" is a mantra will

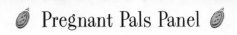

"Will We Ever Pick a Name That Is Meaningful to Both of Us?"

"My husband and I have been going through every baby-name book ever published, I think, and we still haven't come up with anything really personal and meaningful. How can we think of something that will mean a lot to both my husband and me?"

—No Name in Nebraska

Dear No Name,

Your perfect, personal name could very well come from a life-defining experience you've had, something that changed you forever. Let me tell you how we came up with our son's name.

I was happy when our first baby, Nick, was born because then we could seriously contemplate what had always been my dream: to fill our home with lots of adopted children. Don't get me wrong—I loved our son dearly. Plus I was glad for my husband that he would have the "fruit of his loins." But when I was sixteen, I had a vivid dream that lingered with me for weeks. In the dream there was a four-year-old girl from a foreign country who had been sexually abused and needed a loving, healing home. For weeks I would think of the dream and cry, my longing to help this child was so intense. I took the dream to mean that God's purpose for me on earth was to love unloved kids, specifically to adopt and love them as my own.

To first enter into the realm of adoption, my husband, Mike, and I became involved in hosting children from other countries who needed heart surgery in America. Kera was our first little angel. From St. Kitts in the West Indies, Kera was just ten months old when she came to us, and we loved her like a daughter. Alesya from Belarus and Puujee from Mongolia followed, and we both found immense fulfillment in caring for these special children. Meanwhile, we kept waiting for God to open the doors for adoption. But we soon discovered He had other plans for us.

When Nick was about a year old, Mike and I sensed God was leading us to have another biological child. I resisted this with all my might—first by ignoring Him and then, when He couldn't be ignored any longer, by reasoning that the more birth kids we had, the less room we would have for all the others I wanted to adopt.

Well, despite our attempts to prevent it, God won and I became pregnant. The first several months were very difficult because I was so sick. Friends had to come over and care for our son because I couldn't even get out of bed. I just prayed for strength to get through each day.

In the midst of everything, I felt betrayed by God. I knew my attitude grieved the Lord, so one night I asked some friends to come and pray for me. God really spoke to me that night. He showed me that, as beautiful as adoption is, it didn't become necessary until sin entered the world. But pregnancy was given in the very beginning of time as a gift from the Creator.

Suddenly, I realized that I had been looking at adoption as the only gift, but it never occurred to me to receive pregnancy as a blessing, too. I know that sounds ridiculous because the vast majority of people think the other way around, thinking that carrying a child inside of you is the ultimate prize. For me, though, this pregnancy had just felt like something difficult to endure. That night, I realized what a precious gift I had growing inside me.

When we found out I was carrying another boy, I can't even explain the feelings of excitement and love for this little guy that welled up inside me. We wanted his name to reflect the spiritual growth that God had brought about in my life during my pregnancy. So we chose Jonathan—"gift of God"—and Elijah—"God's strength." When he was born, we shortened Jonathan to "Nate," but to us, our wonderful baby son is living up to the combined meanings of his name: "God's gift of strength."

—BECKIE BUWALDA, 29, MOTHER OF NICK, 3, AND NATE, 2

find a wealth of name ideas in other books that have changed their lives. Recently, I came across a lover of all things literate who dubbed his son Yeats in honor of the poet. Friends conferred the Shakespearean name Ariel on their daughter. I know more than one young woman who never forgot the adventures of the irrepressible red-haired orphan from Prince Edward Island, Anne of Green Gables: They gave their daughters the middle or first name Anne. My own name, Lorilee, is rooted in my mom's childhood penchant for reading the Bobbsey twins books by Laura Lee Hope.

Dusting Off Uncle Mortimer

Not long after the relatives learn about the soon-to-be newest member of their clan, expect the issue of family names to arise if not between the two of you then almost definitely from well-meaning kinfolk. "I heard that the old classics are coming back," Aunt Mildred will intone meaningfully, while Dad is suddenly lamenting the good old days when firstborn sons were named after their grandfathers.

Appropriating a family name can be a double-edged sword. Doing so will honor a beloved and admired relative, but you also run the risk of alienating other family members. Even if you and your mate agree that you want to pay tribute to his grandfather, whom you both know and love and whose name you truly like, your family may feel slighted because your long-gone grandpa is being left out. Then the pressure will be on for Boy Number Two to get harnessed with "Herman."

Using family names is fashionable these days for two reasons, according to Pamela Satran, coauthor with Linda Rosenkrantz of *The Last Word on First Names* and *Beyond Jennifer and Jason, Madison and Montana.* Today's couples want to pack their baby's name with as much meaning as possible. Even the middle name, once a freebie slot filled with a short name such as Lynn or John is the cause of much consideration. And Aunt Mildred is right: The old faithful names from the early part of the century are being taken out of the cedar chest, dusted off, and used again for the great-grandchildren of the original Sadies and Sams.

Names which formerly seemed covered in mothballs "begin to come back when young parents who are having babies don't remember anyone else living with that name," says Cleveland Kent Evans, a professor of Psychology at Bellevue University in Bellevue, Nebraska, who writes frequently about baby names. "At that point they start to sound pleasantly old-fashioned rather than ugly and wrinkled. This is usually 110 years after the name hit its previous high point."

 BabyNames.com

For fun and possibly some good ideas, log on to BabyNames. com or another baby-name Web site and try their personalized baby-naming service. You will fill out a short questionnaire about what kinds of names you like (family names, cultural names, and so on) and their staff will come up with several possibilities for you. You may not like their ideas, but who knows?

"I call them the Grandma and Grandpa names," says Satran. "Formal and antiquated names like Harriet and Frances, which have a reverse kind of chic. They are so out there, so kind of ugly they are almost pretty. Like shoes with round toes. At first you say 'ugh,' but then they start to grow on you."

Case in point: My husband's cousin named her baby girl Adeline to honor her own mother, who had given birth to her late in life and who had recently died. Now, little Adeline may not like her name in first grade, when Brianna and Hayley and Madison and Michaela are considered "cool." But her mom has given her a real and rare gift, a name imbued with richness, memories, love, and a deeply meaningful reference. She has truly given her daughter an heirloom.

So scope out your family tree for the brightest and the best. Find a relative whose legacy deserves a namesake. You simply can't do better than that for the newest branch.

Naming Your Dutch/Polish/Peruvian Baby

"Like geodes or fossils, names are intricate, sensual articles full of history and texture," writer Mimi Read said in *Martha Stewart Baby* magazine. Another way to enhance your baby's name with history and texture is by choosing a savory designation that evokes your or your husband's nationality. Most couples represent an intricate mosaic of ethnic backgrounds, and you may want your baby's name to reflect one or more cultures. The Freires (Paulo is a native of Brazil, Lisa is Irish/Italian) have gone back and forth on the cultural issue. "It would be nice for the name to reflect Paulo's heritage because we aren't living in Brazil," Lisa says. "We really want to keep that culture alive for our child, even living here."

Though Lisa sincerely wants to find a Brazilian name for their baby, she hasn't been attracted to any suggested by Paulo and his family so far. He was enthusiastic about Pilar, a Spanish name, but Lisa disliked the ethnic pronunciation of "Pee-lar." Both liked Caleb for a boy, but were turned off by the Portuguese inflection, which rendered the name "Cahleb-ay."

My friend John is Mexican, and his wife is from a German/Welsh

 An Atherton by Any Other Name...

Young couples also have a new option for honoring their fathers, brothers, uncles, and grandfathers: bestowing a traditionally male name on a baby girl. According to Satran, it's the wave of the future. "We [she and Rosenkrantz] forecasted masculine names for girls, and I really see it happening more and more. There is a moving from androgynous names, like Jordan and Taylor, to Kevin and Ryan—just regular boys names." Actress Holly Robinson Peete recently gave her girl twin the name Ryan Elizabeth. Similarly, Teri Hatcher called her daughter Emerson Rose, and Don Johnson plowed new ground with Atherton Grace (she goes by Gracie).

background. They dubbed their third son Zane Mateo to honor his ethnicity. Other friends Joe (born Guiseppe) and his wife Laurie boldly gave their children an extra-firm grip on their Italian heritage with names wonderfully redolent of the Old Country: Francesco, Mario, and Aviana. Michael and his wife, Susan, both of Dutch extraction, opted for Klaas, Anika, and Willem, true-blue Netherlander names.

You may compromise by choosing a name from one tradition for the first name and tying the middle name to another ethnic group in your backgrounds. And remember that the baby's surname makes an ethnic statement in itself. Pamela Satran and her husband, whose last name is Czech, chose Irish names reflecting her ethnicity, leaving their children's last name to represent their father's background.

Mad About Mabel

Whether you choose to believe it or not, television greatly influences culture and, subsequently, names. Many young parents who have never paused their remote control on *Days of Our Lives* would be shocked to learn that their little Kayla's name originated in the mid-to-late eighties as the name of a character on that program.

"Sometimes those TV baby names kind of have an influence again after the reference has receded from people's memories," Satran says. "A great example of this is how the name Kelsey came from *LA Law*. [Characters] Stuart and Ann adopted a baby. They named her Kelsey, which was Ann's last name. It was a completely individual name at the time. Now Kelsey is in the top twenty, and nobody, I'm sure, remembers this was a TV baby name."

One eagerly anticipated baby name in television history was the choice of television's *Mad About You* pair, Paul and Jamie Buchman. The fictitious couple chose Mabel, a name that managed to sound musty, nerdy, and quirky all at once. Many viewers didn't like the name at first, but after a full season of hearing it over and over, the public relaxed toward Baby Buchman's eccentric name.

Could playgroups of the not-too-distant future be populated with Mabels? It is a possibility, predicts Evans. "The first people to revive such a name (as Mabel) are always highly educated, artsy parents, just like the writers for television shows," he notes. "Mabel was a particularly appropriate choice for these writers: One of the sound patterns which is really popular in 'new' names among American parents are names which have the long-A vowel in the first syllable, such as Kayla, Taylor, and Hayley."

The Happy Ending

A few weeks later the Freires still haven't come up with a name, but they are narrowing the list. At the moment, they have tentatively settled on the name Aily, an Irish name they heard at a Celtic music concert. Like them, you are probably finding that the road to naming your baby is long and winding, with points of interest and pitfalls along the way.

Whatever you do, though, don't share your picks too freely because the masses will feel compelled—and justified—in giving their raw opinion. Karenna Gore Schiff and her husband ran into funny looks and less-than-thrilled comments when they were trying to name their firstborn son: "We didn't actually settle on the name Wyatt until the night of his birth. At first we liked the name Wyeth, but it sounded too much like Wyatt with a lisp. After going over and over the long list of names, we landed once again, on Wyatt," she told ThatGlow.com. "I can't reveal what the runner-ups or girl's names were—we may need to save them for later. I have learned that the politics of baby naming can be dangerous. My advice is to keep it to yourself!" And this is a woman who, as her father's daughter, knows about politics.

So zip your lips and don't pay any mind to those who think they can name your baby better than you can! There is, however, one rather huge exception to this rule: If a casual name critic (and remember to always deeply consider the source) mentions that your intended name is too popular, that the daycare she works in already has seven tots running around with this name, for heaven's sake, listen!

I know most of you don't want your baby to stick out like a sore thumb with a social identity that either labels her as weird or squarely smacks a "Kick Me" sign on his forehead. (Fatima and Percival should be avoided.) Names do project images that will follow your child through life, provoking certain expectations on the part of others. Names hint of a personality, even a destiny. I know that, because of her bold and uncompromising

---

 Baby Names from the Great Books

- *Classic-Name Lovers:* Charles (Dickens), Laura (Ingalls Wilder), Julia (Shakespeare), Alice (Walker, in Wonderland), Samuel (Beckett, Longhorne Clemens, Coleridge Taylor), Anna (Karenina), Arthur (the King)

- *Top-Twenty Types:* Emily (Dickinson), Emma (Jane Austen), Jordan *(The Great Gatsby)*, Madeline (from the classic French children's books), Nicholas (Nickelby), Austen (Jane), and Dylan (Thomas)

- *"Goldilocks" Baby Names* (not too hot, not too cold): Lucy *(Mansfield Park)*, Chloe (Longis), and Lily *(To the Lighthouse, Woolf)*, Tess (of the D'Urbervilles), Owen, Nathaniel (Hawthorne), Sebastian *(Tempest, Twelfth Night)*

- And for those willing to scale mountain peaks and dredge the deepest rivers (or just go out on a limb) for a peerless name for their peerless progeny: Gulliver (of Travels fame), Atticus *(To Kill a Mockingbird)*, Truman (Capote), Yeats, Esmé (from the short story by J. D. Salinger, "For Esmé with Love and Squalor"), Eliot (for a girl, to honor T. S. Eliot), Flannery (O'Connor), and Harper (Lee, *To Kill a Mockingbird*)

move, my friend's daughter Zion Esther will have vastly different expectations in life than an Ashley Marie will.

Bottom line: You can do better for your baby than just picking some pleasant, nonoffensive name off the top ten list. Mark my words, Jessica, Brittany, and Michaela are the Amy, Lisa, and Becky of tomorrow. (Have you noticed how many of the stories and quotes in this book are by women named Amy, Lisa, and Becky? That's because I know three Amys, four Lisas, and three Beckys!) Remember this: When they lose their spark of originality, the trendiest names lose everything.

Still, if you have been infatuated with the name Brianna since you were twelve and that is the only name you could ever possibly for your daughter, go right ahead. The main thing is that you love the name!

Whether you opt for a family jewel, a designation infused with ethnic flavor, or a handle as old and durable as the Ten Commandments, one thing is for sure: When you look into your child's wee face for the first time, all the time spent laughing and arguing over the perfect name will be worth every minute.

"This Is Your Brain.
This Is Your Brain on Progesterone."

In her latter days of gestation, Leanne left her purse on top of her car and then drove away, completely unaffected by the frantic motioning of an onlooker in the next car. "I saw this guy waving his arms and pointing to the top of the car, and all I could think of was 'What is wrong with that guy?' Later I realized he was trying to warn me." Not only were Leanne's credit cards, cash, checkbook, driver's license, and the rest of her life inside her purse, but she also had a ruby bracelet inside, a very special gift from her husband, Angel.

The purse showed up a week later in a dollar store on the other side of town, empty except for her ID. For Leanne, and most of us in the latter stages of pregnancy, it's easy to wonder if we might be losing our minds. Well, according to new research, we just might be. British researchers used an MRI to scan the brains of ten moms-to-be during their last trimesters and again a few months after their babies were born. Their discovery? Brain cell volume shrinks during pregnancy, only to plump up again sometime after delivery. Another study conducted by a University of Southern California psychologist found that women also suffer from impaired cognitive function while pregnant, with neither their short-term memories nor their concentration and ability to retain new information working up to par.

This doesn't come as a shock to Doyle, who is plotting ways to attach my keys to my person in a semipermanent way. I don't know why he's so bugged. I only lost two sets of keys. Okay, so it was during a two-day span—and one set turned up ten days later in his hunting backpack! I'm blaming the hound dog for that one.

Then there was the teeny matter of the bagel bag melting to the toaster as I stood and stared at it, waiting for my morning bagel and wondering what that burning smell was. Or the incident of the half-full coffee cup, sitting on the top shelf of the hall closet. Or the episode of ice cream in the pantry, liquefying amid cans of kidney beans and boxes of Jell-O.

I've never been what you might call a clear-headed person, especially in the A.M., but this was kind of extreme.

No one knows exactly what it is that renders an expectant mom's mind to schmaltz (which, if you're wondering, is actually Yiddish for "lard"). Researchers guess that hormones (*and,* I would add, colossal preoccupation and habitual lack of sleep!) cause the incredible shrinking brain phenomenon.

But many late-trimester moms-to-be do report cases of ditziness that range from the above kinds of slips to forgetting their own phone numbers. Thankfully science is now backing up our claims of brain loss, but how can we cope in a world where losing purses and keys leads to no end of new hassles? By pretending you are in the early stages of dementia and taking appropriate measures. Make lists, leave yourself notes, and keep a death grip on those keys. Most importantly, though, cut yourself some slack. After all, says writer Leah Hennen, "Pregnancy has a way of reminding you that there's more at stake than picking up your dry cleaning or beating your husband at Trivial Pursuit—like growing, giving birth to, and being responsible for a brand new life."[1]

Plus, pregnancy is a great excuse for being a bit of an airhead. Use it in good health and remember that this, too, shall pass.

Dream a Little Dream of Me

First your husband is dressed like Barney Rubble. Then you are hugging your high-school boyfriend. Now you're trying to make a quick getaway—on your twelve-year-old nephew's scooter. Zipping down the sidewalk, you have a nagging feeling that you've forgotten something. Suddenly you remember: You left your baby in the soup aisle!

Have you lost your mind? No—not your waking mind anyway. During pregnancy, your dreams take on a new intensity, zaniness, and sometimes significance. In her book *Pregnancy and Childbirth*, Tracie Hotchner writes, "Dreams have an important function at this time in your life. Think of them as messages, information about yourself that you have no other way of finding out. Dreams are things to discuss, ideas to recognize."[2]

If your dreams seem nuttier than usual—filled with talking cows, long-forgotten crushes, and dead relatives very much alive and well (and wearing garish jewelry)—blame the progesterone gushing through your veins along with your alternating thrills and terrors about pregnancy and motherhood. Talk about Technicolor! Joseph and his seven fatted calves seem tame in comparison to some of the neon images that pop up in a pregnant woman's sleep. Since Joseph's not currently available to offer his two cents about the significance of your p.g. dreams, it's a good thing many of these mini mind-flicks are easy enough to figure out.

Here's another reason your dream life has shifted into high gear: If you're waking up during the night to pee, ease a leg cramp, or shift to a more comfy position, you're likely to interrupt a dream-filled cycle of REM sleep.

If you're anything like me—and loads of pregnant pals past and present—these dreams you're suddenly aware of are a bit alarming, especially if you're not used to them. I do believe in paying some attention to our dreams, which I once heard described as the inner part of your mind trying to talk to the outer part. But I'm not saying you need to begin a dream journal or that every little snippet of your dreams needs to be psychoanalyzed, yet by being mindful you might learn a thing or two about yourself.

"In the state of heightened awareness that pregnancy provides, the dreaming cycle itself can become an invaluable asset for a mother-to-be, like clues to a newly discovered treasure map," writes Raina M. Paris, author of *The Mother-to-Be's Dream Book*.[3]

So whether you're already an avid dream-fiend who revels in flying dreams and jots down every plot detail of every narcoleptic reverie, or whether you usually can't recall a thing when you wake up, here's an unofficial guide to those crazy mommy-to-be dreams:

The Nifty Nine
Dream Themes

1. The Funhouse Dreams

Enjoy your all-new, digitally enhanced, groovy dream world! Dreams are like funhouse mirrors that reflect what's going on in your real life. If in your pre-preggers days the picture was a little fuzzy, now you should be able to tune in to some wild and woolly nocturnal programming. Sometimes dreams exceed our imaginations and really take us on a magic carpet ride. If you're one of the lucky ones who have flying dreams, have fun and hold on to that soaring feeling during your earthbound days.

2. Leaving-the-Baby-Somewhere Dreams

It doesn't take Carl Jung to get to the bottom of the abandoning-Baby dream. Forgetting your precious bundle at the grocery store, the gym, the car, or the hospital in your sleep doesn't mean you're going to do that in real life. Experts say this is a huge theme in the dreams of pregnant women, who are worried on some level that they may not be mommy material after all. "Being unprepared, losing things, forgetting to feed the baby, losing car keys or even the baby can express the fear of not being adequate to the task of motherhood," say the authors of *What to Expect When You're Expecting*. Such dreams may provide a way for your subconscious to deal with any fears and insecurities you no doubt have about pregnancy and impending motherhood. I dreamed this particular dream even more often during my second pregnancy as I wondered if I could handle the demands of a toddler and a newborn. The *What to Expect* ladies also weigh in on a few more typical dream themes:

3. Attack Dreams

Being attacked or hurt may represent your sense of vulnerability.

4. Trapped-in-a-Cave Dreams

Being trapped in a tight space may indicate the fear of being figuratively tied down. Dreaming that you're running away, falling from a great height, or trapped in a room may express your concern about losing the freedom of your pre-baby days.

5. Death-and-Resurrection Dreams

The *What to Expect* authors add, "Lost parents and other relatives reappearing—may be the subconscious mind's way of linking old and new generations." Okay, that one's a little bizarre, but I include it because one night while pregnant with Ezra I had the most amazing, beautiful dream about my beloved Grandma, who died almost four years earlier. In it she was vibrantly healthy, almost youthful looking, and so happy to see me. I woke up feeling enriched, as if I had spent time with one of my favorite people.

6. Not-so-Pretty-Woman Dreams

Is the you of your dreams unappealing? "Becoming unattractive or repulsive to your husband expresses nearly every woman's fear that pregnancy will destroy her looks," they write.[4] Also, related to this fear are:

7. Sex Dreams

Erotic dreams, writes Patricia Garfield, author of *Women's Bodies, Women's Dreams*, are more likely the larger the mother-to-be gets; they tend to occur most often during the final three months of pregnancy. "The reasons for erotic dreams in the pregnant woman are as varied as the women themselves. Nevertheless, most mothers-to-be share a concern about their changing figure and its effect on their sex life. Intercourse is necessarily more awkward during the final months of pregnancy. Deprived of her accustomed regularity or intensity of sex, the expectant mother sometimes compensates for it in dreams," she writes. "Beyond whatever physical deprivation they may feel, pregnant women often feel insecure about their continued attractiveness to men. Gripping furniture for support in raising or seating herself, her ankles swollen, the mother-to-be finds her body increasingly difficult to maneuver. Erotic dreams during pregnancy simply offer the comforting reassurance, 'Don't worry. You see, you are sexy, alluring, and lovable.'"[5]

8. Freaky-Baby or Gender-Bender Dreams

If you dream that your baby is deformed, that he or she is a giant or a troll or has some other freakish quality, you're not alone. Many women have these nightmares, especially in their last trimester when it's normal to worry about your baby's health (see chapter 8). If you wake up in a cold sweat, agonizing over your dream, take a deep breath, pray for perspective on your dream, and ask God to give you His peace about your baby's well-being.

If you have been dreaming of tiny tutus and toe shoes, and you don't know the sex of your child, your dreams may express a deep preference for one sex over another. Or maybe something else is happening. Janet Jones Gretzky had a dream that confirmed the actual sex of her child: "At 14 weeks we were told we were having a girl. I bought the little dresses," she told *Fit Pregnancy* magazine. "Then the night before we had the ultrasound at 18 weeks, I had this vivid dream that we were having a boy. I saw the penis. And guess what? It's a boy."[6] Again, pray it through, and ask God to give you a desire for a healthy baby above all, regardless of gender.

9. Symbolic Dreams

This just cracks me up, but you never know, right? In her book, Paris analyzes a bunch of dream symbols—everything from acorns to yoga, ovens to vegetables. This "symbol" caught my eye: "Whale: If you are in your last trimester you might be feeling like a great whale. The whale is also a powerful symbol for the female creative energy of life and a clue as to how big a deal this pregnancy really us. The size, color, and demeanor of this great mammal, as well as your reaction to the dream, are other clues for you to consider."[7] She's right on one count at least! One does feel whalish in the third trimester, more the blue whale variety than the puny beluga. And if you happen to be carrying a son whom you plan to call Jonah, as I was the first time around, double that huge marine mammal feeling!

What to Do This Month

☐ Buy or borrow baby-name books.

☐ Nest: If you're going to sew curtains or what-have-you for the baby's room, get going on any sewing/painting (in a well-ventilated room)/needlepoint/crafty types of projects.

☐ Keep long-distance friends and family involved in your experience. Send copies of the ultrasound pictures, photos of your burgeoning belly, and details of your pregnancy—like how often the baby is moving, to bridge the miles.

☐ If you're a scrapbooky sort, decide if you want a regular or special baby scrapbook. Order it and start cropping ultrasound and pregnancy pics.

☐ Journal idea: This month, you may know if you're having a boy or girl. Tell him or her how you felt at hearing the news as well as your hopes and dreams for your son or daughter. Be sure to jot down for posterity the often-hilarious process of coming up with a name. Someday your child will think it's fascinating to know which names were up for consideration and why!

Dear P or E,

C'mon now, little girl (or guy), give your old mother a break and move a little less. By the feel of it, you've got a mini-Olympics of your very own going on inside my belly: aerial skiing, the luge, triple salchows—ei yi yi! I mean, that's great if you're athletic and all, but save the stunts for *aprés* birth, okay?

It's October, my favorite month, and the leaves on the trees are a glorious riot of orange, yellow, and, my favorite, maple-leaf red. So how did you like your second trip to Canada, the "True North Strong and Free"? I am so glad we decided to go to Tante Susie and Uncle Witold's anniversary at the last minute. Oma and Opa were there, and lots of my aunts and uncles and cousins. Uncle Dan and Aunt Tina were there too, and Aunt Tina's not even showing! We got to soak in all the Canadiana, especially the moving coverage of Pierre Trudeau's funeral. I'm sure by the time you read this, you will have heard the story of how I met him when I was just a little girl.

You and Jonah are both Americans and Canadians, and it will be exciting to see how you integrate the strengths of each country into your own worldview. Daddy's a Baptist and I'm a Mennonite; he's a country boy and I'm a city girl. There are so many varied ideas and views and passions for you to choose from! You may be more like one of us or totally, indisputably you. We can't wait to find out! Stay cool in there, baby mine.

Love,
Mama

Stretchy Pants, Sleeplessness, and One Sticky Topic

The history of man for the nine months preceding his birth would probably be far more interesting, and contain events of greater moment, than all the threescore and ten years that follow it.
—SAMUEL TAYLOR COLERIDGE

Snapshot! Baby's getting bigger, and so are you. Your little one may have topped three pounds, but you may have added twenty to thirty. Your baby is smiling, frowning, scrunching up her wee nose, and basically testing out all the bells and whistles on her face. She may be crying, although no one is sure why in utero babes shed a few tears. That rhythmic little beat is your daughter hiccuping like a tiny drum majorette. If your ribs start to feel a bit stepped on, or kicked, or poked, chances are she has flipped head over heels and is in the head-down position, where she'll stay until birth.

Friends Don't Let Friends Wear Tents

About eight years ago, my sister-in-law Jodi said something shocking to me. She had recently learned that she was pregnant with her third baby, who turned out to be our adorable nephew Ryan. Mind you, this was years before pregnancy was remotely a consideration in my own life, and the whole process seemed as distant and exotic as Bora Bora. Anyway, she told me that she and her husband Mike were going to celebrate by shopping for stretch pants and roomy tops. "Mike just loves the way I look in maternity clothes," she said. Wow! In our thin-obsessed culture, to know that her love truly admired her swelling form was no doubt a marvelous gift for Jodi.

I must admit to you here and now that I am a certifiable clotheshorse. I love flipping through glossy fashion magazines trying to figure out how the flamboyant, theatrical garments of the runways could possibly translate into a normal woman's wardrobe. But over the years my penchant for sartorial splendor has, of course, clashed more often than not with the lack of copious amounts of cash. I've had to learn to scope out cute stuff on the cheap.

Pregnancy, though, is a season of life in which just basic dressing is difficult, never mind garbing your ballooning body with a modicum of flair. If you live someplace where there are four seasons, maternity dressing is even trickier. And assembling a pregnancy wardrobe without gouging your checkbook is, in fact, rocket science.

One thing to be thankful for: maternity clothes are much cuter than they used to be. In the days when Lucy Ricardo was expecting Little Ricky, she wore this voluminous, polka-dot tent with a mammoth bow tie and Peter Pan collar—on television. That thing is probably in the Smithsonian now, and I'm happy to report no fashion designers seem eager to revive it.

"Until a few years ago, the driving philosophy behind maternity clothes seemed to be to hide the pregnancy and draw attention away from the belly and up to the pregnant woman's glowing face," writes Vicki Iovine in *The Girlfriend's Guide to Pregnancy*. "Putting together most maternity outfits involved gathering together yards and yards of fabric, invariably some sort of polyester, up around the poor pregnant woman's neck and letting it skirt out to a circumference of about twenty feet."[1]

The first trimester should be the easiest unless this is not your first pregnancy. In that case, your pants may not zip up very easily, very early on. Usually you can just keep on wearing your normal clothes until Weeks Twelve to Fourteen or so. If you have to buy a bunch of new stuff for, say, a vacation or something, bite the bullet and buy a size up. You and I both know you're a size 10, but Baby may not, and you'll appreciate that size 12 dress when it glides over your expanding waistline/hips/etc. This is also not the time to buy a lot of trendy outfits with the thought that they will fit you again next year. *That's a big "if," honey.* Not only do you have no earthly idea how fast your postpregnancy pounds will say adieu, but fashion changes so fast that this year's fad is sure to be next year's folly. Another first trimester trick: the rubber band. Loop a rubber band through the buttonhole on your pants or jeans and fasten it to the button to gain a few more weeks' use.

The second trimester usually presents the biggest challenge. "This is the sticky wicket of maternity dressing because in the fourth or fifth months you may be too small for the full-blown tummy pockets and too large for nearly everything else in your closet," writes Iovine.[2] Well said. With my first pregnancy, I popped out at about sixteen weeks. This one? Let's just say the popping came sooner and leave it at that.

My first shopping expedition lead me to Target, a truly excellent source of stylish and affordable maternity wear. It was July, and I had inarguably run out of anything decent to wear for any occasion. So, even though only two months—tops—of heat remained in Michigan's summer, I was forced to pile up my cart with capri pants, shorts, T-shirts, and summer dresses. In my mind, I was a solid medium-sized gal, and although the medium clothes looked a tad small, I felt sure I could pull it off and get some good use out of them. Little did I know I would expand from a medium to a large before two months were up. The upshot of this story? I only got about six weeks out of almost every article of clothing I bought that day. The weather got too chilly for some stuff, and my body got too big for others. The moral? "If you buy too early, you buy too small," Liz Lange, designer and owner of Liz Lange maternity told *In Style* magazine.[3]

So be proactive and buy big. The worst that can happen is you have some extra fabric floating around your form. This, my friend, is a far superior scenario to having your button holes strain valiantly against the burden of a size large belly in a size medium casing (yes, I said "casing," as in sausage).

The good news of the third trimester is that no one thinks you've been spending quality time at the smorgasbord. You look pregnant—and if you don't, we don't want to know about it! The bad news is you are probably going to run out of things to wear. Both of my third trimesters came when the people of Michigan were enthralled with fall. My capri pants still fit, but I would have frozen my ankles off had I worn them. So it was back to the maternity store for more clothes.

Yes, it was hard to justify buying a bunch of new garments when I only had a few months to wear them. But ask any pregnant woman who has stayed home from an outing just because she has nothing suitable to wear—you gotta have a few things on hand. In addition to some staples (see this month's Nifty Nine), I bought a vivid, zippy sweater and a fun pink stretchy shirt just to perk things up a bit. At thirty-seven weeks, most of my big sweatshirts (even the huge ones) didn't really fit anymore, so I alternated between a couple of maternity sweaters almost every single day.

One morning—laundry day, incidentally, which pinches the clothing shortage even more—I was forced to wear an odd assemblage, part pajama/part plus-size bargain T-shirt bought the previous summer, two pieces which didn't match by any stretch of the imagination. But at least my belly wasn't hanging out. Now Doyle thinks that's a cute look, but in fact it made me look like a cross between a hobo clown and a Weeble (remember, they wobble but they don't fall down). At this point, your motto should be "coverage, coverage, coverage." And remember, you don't have to last that much longer.

The Nifty Nine
Ways to Marvelous Maternity Dressing

1. Buy the Staples at the Maternity Store

Vicki Iovine suggests that the following are maternity wear essentials: bathing suit, leggings, bras, panties, and jeans. I would add to this list overalls, which pull off the slick trick of being usable with your pre-partum shirts, tops, turtlenecks, and so on. Of all the items in my pregnancy wardrobe, I could not have made it without those handy dandy overalls.

2. Black is Beautiful for Anyone
Who Has to Contend with a Few Bulges

Your belly at seven months probably qualifies. Plus black is so chic, so polished that you can avoid looking like an oversized little girl in one of those ubiquitous flowery baby doll tops. If you like, pair some black pants with a bright top for some color.

3. Invest in a Good Bra

Whether you're planning an evening out or an afternoon lolling around the house, you'll look and feel better if your underwear is comfortable. Your breasts may go up by as much as three cup sizes, so look for bras made of 100 percent cotton with wide straps and bands to support growing breast tissue.

4. Beg, Borrow, and Steal Maternity Clothes
from Your Friends and Relatives

Most of your previously pregnant friends and family members will gladly hand over their collection of maternity clothes that is just sitting around the house waiting for their next gestation period. This kind of sharing works especially well with friends whose pregnancies have spanned the same seasons as yours. Not only will this borrowing amplify the slim pickings in your own closets, but also it means expensive maternity clothes won't go to waste. When you're done with your clothes, return the favor either to the same pal who passed her stuff on or to someone else who needs it.

5. Check Out the Secondhand Shops

Even if you've never been much of a thrift-store shopper, now is the time to scour a few consignment and secondhand stores. Many cities have such stores that cater exclusively to pregnant women and their babies. My friend Margaret, the queen of thrift, spotted a pair of maternity jeans in my size at Goodwill. The cost? Twenty-five cents, give or take. And I have worn them about forty times.

6. Celebrate!

You're in rare form, so go on at least one spree, even a little one, and buy something that makes you feel pretty. This doesn't have to be something too fancy or too expensive, just something that fits and makes you feel good.

7. "Wear Fitted Clothes to Show Off Your Beautiful Belly..."

...Nadine Belfort, co-owner of L'Attesa, told *In Style* magazine. "You want to celebrate the pregnancy, not just survive it."[4]

8. Accentuate the Positive

If you've always been a bit vain about your cute knees and thin calves, now is the time to alert the public to their merits. If you've been working out, as has been strongly suggested (hint, hint), wear sleeveless tops and dresses to show off those triceps.

9. Accessorize!

Wear jewelry and scarves. They'll put the attention firmly on your glowing, radiant face. Writer Jennifer Galvin fondly recalls a lovely watch she bought when she was pregnant with her third child: "Finally, something pretty and petite that FIT. What a concept! The poor woman must have thought I was insane as she witnessed my glee. I still wear it to this day. It's special because it reminds me of the beginning—those precious moments I felt my baby growing inside me. It has become a little less sparkly, but no less special."[5]

O For a Thousand Nights to Sleep

One night late in my pregnancy with Ezra I woke up four times, which was a bargain compared to my usual number of nocturnal wakings. In the first place, I couldn't get to sleep until about 1 A.M.—after having chatted with my husband and turned out the lights at 11 P.M. Then I had such a vivid, complex, I-was-there dream that I woke up with a jolt at about 3:30. It was like being in a movie theater when all of a sudden the projector jams, the lights shut off, and everything is shockingly still. Then at 5:00, I had to roll over again because my hipbone was throbbing in pain. I rolled over again at 6:00. At 7:00 my toddler crawled into bed with me and I had to shuffle all kinds of blankets and pillows to accommodate his floppy little form.

That morning I felt, in the quaint words of my cowboy father-in-law, like a horse that's been rode hard and put away wet. And that particular night's string of wake-ups didn't even include the usual slumber-interrupting stumble to the bathroom or my favorite—leg cramps. I'm not whining. Well, I am, but it has a purpose. I'm simply telling you what you already know: In your third trimester, the quality of your sleep reaches an all-time low. Experts say that the majority of women have insomnia and other sleep problems during pregnancy. And studies show that pregnant women in their third trimester have fewer periods of deep sleep and wake up more often during the night.

My friend Amy would toss and turn like a whirling dervish during her first pregnancy, especially between 2 and 4 A.M. During one particularly frustrating night of insomnia, she got up, got dressed, and drove down to the nearest Dunkin' Donuts. A policeman (naturally she would find a policeman in a donut shop!), seeing that she was highly pregnant, approached her with some concern and asked if she was all right. It was the middle of the night after all. Amy assured him that she was fine, that she just had a yen for chocolate donuts. She wasn't finished with her insomniac wanderings either. Seized with a sudden desire to play Scrabble, Amy's next stop was a twenty-four-hour grocery/convenience/all-purpose superstore-type place, where she picked up a new game. Her husband, Steve, eventually woke up and realized that his wife wasn't lying beside him. He found her in the living room, beating herself at Scrabble.

I've never actually left the building during a sleepless night, but I have watched way too many infomercials regaling the benefits of workout machines, food dehydrators, and miracle skin potions. By now you get the message. Getting—and staying—comfortable in bed may be one of your greatest challenges during pregnancy, particularly if you're used to sleeping on your stomach or your back. I can't tell you how much I pined for the days of snoozing with my face smashed into my pillows. (I know, I know. This causes wrinkles and creases and all manner of skin-care chaos, but that's how I love to sleep.)

While stomach sleeping is pretty much impossible, back sleeping can be downright harmful. Sleeping on your back means that your intestines, inferior vena cava (the vein that carries blood from your lower body to the heart), and back must bear the full weight of your heavy uterus. It can also cause backaches, hemorrhoids, inefficient digestion, less-than-optimum breathing and circulation, and even low blood pressure.

Sleeping on your left side benefits your baby by maximizing blood flow and nutrients to the placenta. Apparently the left-side method also helps your kidneys get rid of waste products and fluids, which may help trim down those bloated ankles and feet. But if your right side for some reason works for you, go for it. A few extra nutrients for Baby and a few less layers of puff aren't worth you turning into a sleep-deprived maniac.

A pillow between your legs is comfy, and any old pillow will do. In my opinion, those maternity body pillows are just a lot of fluff. (And my friend Lisa's husband, Tim, said that her sleeping with a body pillow was like having a third person in bed with them!) In your third trimester, experts also suggest wearing a sleeping bra and a maternity belt to give extra "uphold" to your breasts, belly, and back. Sleeping in a bra sounds like extra torture, but the maternity belt thing is worth a try. One night, heaving my massive belly from one side to the other actually caused a strain in my abdominal muscles, which woke me up, naturally. I was on the verge of installing a pulley system from the ceiling, to be frank. Of course, you won't believe this until it happens to you.

Sleep Aids

Chamomile tea is safe to drink during your pregnancy, and it's long been hailed as a soporific. Try a nice warm cup as part of your bedtime routine.

Warm milk boosts the amino acid 1-tryptophan, which may make you drowsy by increasing your serotonin levels.

Ask your mate for a massage, and try a routine of gentle stretching exercises to loosen tense muscles.

Talk to your doc about taking a safe, tested sleep aid. Every physician has a different take on this, but mine gave me the green light to take Benadryl on nights when my insomnia was really bad. Tell your husband you won't be able to operate heavy machinery, like the washing machine and dishwasher. The break from the chores alone should help you snooze!

If lying on your side puts too much pressure on your hips—which it will, no question about it—try one of those egg-carton-shaped layers that goes on top of your mattress and under the sheet. Some pregnant women swear by them.

If frequent bathroom breaks keep you up at night, try not to drink as much during the late afternoon and evening. Doing so will hopefully cut down on the number of nighttime bathroom breaks. Also, experts in such matters suggest you lean forward when you pee, thus completely emptying your bladder.

Heartburn is another foe to a good night's sleep. Blame progesterone, which slackens the valve that separates the esophagus from the stomach, allowing gastric acids to seep back up the pipe, and *voila!*, heartburn. Plus, your growing baby is taking up loads of space that was once used to facilitate digestion. But for you glass-half-full gals (who are swiftly becoming glass-half-empty gals due to chronic lack of sleep), there is a silver lining, such as it is. The same process that causes you discomfort actually benefits your baby: Nutrients that linger in your bloodstream due to slower digestion can be absorbed more fully into your baby's system.

Heartburn is nasty, no doubt about it. So try to minimize it by passing up acidic, spice-laden dishes as well as other well-known culprits like coffee and citrus fruits. Some pregnant pals avoid gum chewing at all costs, especially peppermint, which makes things worse.

"You don't understand, Lorilee. I get heartburn from eating *yogurt!*" I hear you, truly. It seems these days as if nothing goes down the hatch without making a return visit in a more aggressive form. Conventional wisdom proposes eating small, more frequent meals, sleeping with one or two extra pillows under your head and shoulders, and wearing loose clothing (in the event that your pajamas are too tight or something)! My best tip is to have a stash of Rolaids or Tums right by the bed. Or fall asleep with one dissolving in your mouth. Yeah, you *could* do fractions at the blackboard with those chalky-tasting little orbs, but they beat back heartburn like nothing else.

And now, how about those leg cramps? Not only does your back feel the strain of your extra girth, but your legs do too, which is why they sometimes protest in the form of nighttime leg cramps. You can also point a finger at too much phosphorus (found in processed meats, snack foods, and soda) and too little calcium and potassium. One more explanation, should you require one, is that your expanding uterus is sitting squarely on the nerves leading from your trunk to your legs. These third-trimester treats range in intensity from the mildly annoying to the excruciating. Try sleeping through one of these muscular tantrums and then tell me how you pulled it off. Of all the common causes of pregnancy wakeups, this is, in my opinion, the worst.

Sometimes a cramp can be alleviated by simply wiggling and flexing your feet and legs the right way. At other times you have to haul your body out of bed, stand upright, and yelp in pain so loudly that you wake the whole household. I heard of one poor woman who had to stand in her bare feet in the cold garage before hers let up. (At least with leg cramps your husband can relate to the sensation. While it's safe to say he's never experienced lugging a thirty-pound weight on his abdomen or had heartburn after eating pretzels, he's probably had a few charley horses in his lifetime.)

What can you do about it? It goes without saying, start by knocking

 ## God's Night School

The very best thing you can do with all of that extra predawn time is pray. There is a book out there somewhere by Connie Soth called *Insomnia: God's Night School.* I haven't read it, but the great title has stuck with me for years. Those insomniac hours, which really add up, could be put to excellent use (certainly something superior to playing silly alphabet games all night long). Who hasn't struggled to find decent time to pray? In the middle of the night there's nothing to do, everyone is asleep, and you find yourself with an open slot of one, two, or maybe more, hours of time. You can use this time to deepen your relationship with your Father in heaven as you pray for your growing baby, for your new role as a mother, for your husband, your friends, your family—the list of people and situations that need praying for is endless. (See chapter 8 for more on prayer and pregnancy.)

off the Slim Jims and salami. A prebedtime banana milkshake, full of potassium and calcium, could be a sweet, easy preventive measure. Stretch your calf muscles before hitting the sack and wiggle your toes and ankles during the day as you think of it.

In addition to the garden-variety sleep interruptions, there's also plain old insomnia. Not much is worse than watching the numbers on your clock radio change in the middle of the night and knowing that the next morning's toddler chase-a-thon or work meeting will be brutal. Not only do many pregnant women struggle to fall asleep in the first place, but drifting off again after a leg cramp or bathroom break isn't always easy either.

 ## Cha-Ching!

Experts say that Baby may add about $10,000 to your expenses in his first year. This rather shocking number includes insurance copays for birth, immunizations, and doctor visits, formula (about $1,000 per year), diapers, clothes, a stroller, a car seat, and so on. Don't let the dollar amount overwhelm you. Just do your best to manage your money wisely. Baby probably doesn't need a brand new wardrobe from Oilily or Gymboree. And remember to take one day at a time.

So you're up—bright-eyed and bushy tailed. Alive! Awake! Alert! Enthusiastic! It's 3:14 A.M. The catchy pop tune you heard on the radio two days ago (or, worse, the theme from *Sesame Street, Barney,* or *Veggie Tales*) is blaring in your head. An hour later, you contemplate having the blasted ditty surgically removed from your brain. Why can't you have something soothing playing in the radio-of-the-mind? Something like Brahms Lullaby? Too late for that. You begin to obsess about the next day, and how wretched you are going to feel, and how inconvenient that will be since you have so much to do. But your eyes are not even at half-mast. They are blinking at full speed as you count the slats in your miniblinds.

The man of the house is, naturally, snoring cheerfully beside you. You are not finding this helpful in your quest for shuteye, and frankly you are about to smash his vibrating olfactory glands with your pillow.

I have to be honest with you and admit that I've never found many of the conventional sleep remedies—warm milk, progressive muscle relaxation, guided imagery, that kind of thing—to be very helpful. But you might benefit greatly, so go right ahead.

Remember Amy and her Scrabble Solitaire? I have a similar solo game, but this one you can play as you lie there in agony listening to Loverboy's nasal cacophony. It's like Scattergories, but you play in your mind against yourself, see? The beauty of this little game is that is based on the alphabet (not hard to recall at 4 A.M.), and the categories are endless. So pick a subject—say, soft drinks—and just roll with it: Arizona Tea, Bart's Root Beer, Clearly Canadian (double points on that one). If you get stumped, just pass and keep going. Pick an easy category that you know well. Now is not the time to dig deep for trivia from organic chemistry or the Crimean War. It's just good, clean, mindless fun, more interesting than counting sheep and less stimulating than predicting your 401(k) benefits or rehashing a conflict with your best friend. (This also works as a road-trip game, if you're so inclined.)

To Work or Not to Work? The Question of the Hour

Of all the choices you face, one of the most complex, multifaceted, and possibly heartrending is whether you will go out to work or stay at home after your baby arrives. Even if you've always dreamed of being a full-time housewife, various factors may complicate matters. And if you've invested yourself passionately in a job, you may have always had every intention to return to work after your maternity leave. But now that motherhood is really, truly around the corner, you could be having second thoughts.

"When you've just given birth to a sweet new baby, can you happily hand her over to someone else for a good part of every day?" You may be hearing—or asking yourself—this question a lot lately, but the truth is, the issue's all abstract until D-Day and the ensuing weeks and months. My friend Linda spent years in management and watched many new moms come and go. "Most of them say they'll be back when the baby comes, but some of them change their minds—even when they swore they wouldn't—when that baby actually arrives."

 "Don't Miss Your Kids"

Author Lisa Tawn Bergren says that many people told her to not miss her kids. "I used it as a general rule. When I started missing my kids, I made a change. I never wanted to look back and regret what I had chosen. After Olivia was born I cut back to thirty hours a week and worked from home. After Emma was born, I cut back to twenty-one hours a week and continued to work from home. It was another two years before God finally let me go from my 'calling' at work to focus on the three Fs: my own fiction, family, and faith-life."

Other women have for their whole lives imagined themselves as at-home mom types, but when the reality of being at home all day every day sets in, they desperately miss their jobs.

Of course, you may not have a choice if your family depends on your income to pay the bills. But if you do go back to work, what about child-care? Who is going to be there with your child when you are not?

Adding to the confusion—and the guilt—is the range of expert opinions on this subject. Some studies show negative results in children when both parents work full time. Other experts dispute or contradict these findings.

Working moms may feel guilty that they are not caring for their children 24/7, using available free time for baking and educational games. Stay-at-home moms may feel shame that they aren't using their education or worry that money is tight because only their husbands are bringing home a check. Many also complain of feeling isolated, and they long for the more tangible rewards—creative and social as well as financial—that the workplace provides.

One thing is definite: The choice to work outside the home or not is a highly personal one. At the same time it is also a very touchy subject; few people feel neutral on the matter. Yet, it seems to me that each choice is deeply—if not consciously—informed by cultural pressures of one ilk or another. On the one hand you've got a certain camp urging you to achieve, bring home some of that bacon, and reap the rewards of equality in the workplace. Then again you may be feeling pressure from peers, from church, from your parents, from whomever, to conform to their expectations of what good mothering entails.

I've seen women who absolutely thrive in their role as the mommy with the mostest. They find true satisfaction in serving their families full time. Some of these women are called to be stay-at-home mothers, and they are using their God-given gifts in the best possible way. They are good mothers. Others have decided that they have the energy to balance work and family and that, because they are pursuing a vocation they find gratifying, they are happier, saner people. They are good mothers, too.

Don't let anyone tell you what is best for you and your family. After you've prayerfully considered your options, then make a decision and be open to changing your mind as your child grows older. (Sheath those claws, girlfriends!) And try to respect the choices of other young moms. It's so easy to judge without really knowing the needs and pressures and perspectives of another person.

I admit that I have criticized, in my mind at least, working mothers whom I suspect could cut back to part time, but who seem to be working to buy grownup toys. I have also judged friends who seem ill suited to staying at home and who could be doing themselves and their families a world of good by getting a part-time job. I'm working on not judging. In fact, the longer I'm a mom, the clearer it seems to me that we all face our own unique challenges. The main thing to do is to support each other in the monumental job of parenting.

Reads of the Month

How to Raise a Family on Less Than Two Incomes: The Complete Guide to Managing Your Money Better So You Can Spend More Time with Your Kids by Denise Topolnicki

The Financial Peace Planner by Dave Ramsey

Subscribe to *Working Mother* magazine if you plan on continuing your job. It's filled with ideas for money management and how to make career and family work.

Besides, you have more than two choices. Working for a paycheck doesn't have to be all-or-nothing. Use your noodle and cook up a creative way of making your own rules. You can work full time or stay home full time. You can work part time or work at home. Job sharing is also worth considering. Maybe your employer will work with you to develop a plan that benefits you both. As the pregnant pals who weighed in below will testify, great rewards await those who think outside the box a little bit, especially on a complicated issue like this. In light of that point, consider one more possibility: Think about whether or not your husband could be the full-time parent. According to Oprah.com, some two million men in the United States are stay-at-home dads. My friend Nancy is a bond trader who works full time. Her husband, Mince, stays at home with their daughter, Eva, while pursuing his education degree part time. John is another at-home dad who cares for his two school-age kids while their mom tends to patients in her medical practice. Even if you don't happen to have a job that's higher paying and has better benefits than your mate, he may be more suited to the daily domestic grind than you are. (And let's just drop the "Mr. Mom" comments, shall we? Puh-lease.)

"I Can't Decide Whether to Stay Home or Return to Work."

"I work full time at an advertising agency, and I do enjoy my job. I have always thought I would stay at home when we started having kids, but now that I'm pregnant, I don't know what to do. How did you come to your decision about whether or not you would work?"

—ON-THE-FENCE IN OKLAHOMA

(For this PPP, I asked four pals to give us a peek into their decision-making process. Each one is a fabulous mother, and I know they all put hours of thought and prayer into their decisions.)

Why I Decided to Work at Home

My decision to work from home was one of the easiest and most natural to make. The transition wasn't as easy, but my husband, Ray, and I have sensed God's leading since I moved from the computer at work to the computer at home.

I was working full time when our first daughter was born and continued to work after the second came along. That choice was out of necessity, but Ray and I both felt it was the right one. During a job switch, however, I began to sense God was leading me home. I enjoyed my work, but I began to realize that it couldn't be the most important thing in my life. Then Ray was offered a nearly full-time teaching position. This was wonderful, but I still needed to work. That year was one of the most difficult we'd ever experienced.

Our oldest daughter was in kindergarten, and our youngest was in daycare all day. Ray and I both realized that, while the extra money was nice, it didn't make up for the stress, fatigue, and time away from our children. That year taught me what's really important in life: God and family.

When Ray was offered a full-time position, I turned in my resignation. I decided to pursue freelance writing for several reasons. One is that I

(continued on next page)

can work around the children's schedules. Our two daughters are in school all day, and now we have two preschool age boys. I can write when they nap, at midnight, or while they are trashing the house.

Second, the extra money is helpful. It allows us to build our savings account, take modest vacations, and not feel so strapped each month. We choose to live on one income, but my freelance money takes the edge off.

Third, I think it's important to use the gifts and talents God has given me. If God can use me in the area of writing, then I need to be writing. But attention to God's timing is an important part of this. My priority has got to be my family, but if God wants to use me for other things as well I need to be open.

Finally, I work from home because I like it. I enjoy what I do. I get to interview people, write, read, and surf the Internet wearing slippers and no makeup. What more could I want?

—ANN BYLE, MOTHER OF BREE, 10, ABBY, 9, JAY, 3, AND JARED, 1

Why I Decided to Work Full Time

Sometimes I wonder myself! There are days when my son wakes up and needs me to be at home. There are days when I'm worn down from keeping on top of my job and the house, keeping a marriage alive and helping a child feel loved and secure. I feel stress like you do. I worry about childcare like you do.

Yet when I find myself at the proverbial end of my rope, I know, deep down, that I will always feel the need to work. Ask my friends, ask my husband, ask my sister. I'm of the conviction that God gave me a talent for a reason and I need to glorify Him by using it. Yet He also gave me a beautiful child, and if the work stint begins to wreck havoc on our lives, a change may have to occur. So for right now I work as a marketing manager of a Christian publishing company. It thrills me to know that the books we are producing help people in every aspect of their lives.

Advice: If you make the decision to work, choose a job you love. If you don't love it, you're not doing yourself, your family, or your employer any favors.

My mom works. Maybe that's why I know that it can turn out okay. She was (and still is) an elementary school teacher. She loves it. She's good at it. Throughout my childhood, she was still my mom. I learned from her example, adapting some of her strategies for making it work and also developing my own.

But I couldn't do this at all if it weren't for my husband. He has supported me from day one, saying that he knows my personality and knows that I need that outlet of work. From the time I started back after my maternity leave, we made a point of making sure that our time at home with Zach was quality. We set aside chores until he went to bed, and we devoted the evening to him. Now that he's older, he "helps" us with jobs that need to be done (like shoveling snow or doing laundry), spending time with us but learning as well. And of course, we love to play! We also don't go out much individually or as a couple during the week because those evenings are dedicated to our family.

Great childcare is a must, of course. And there are gems out there. Zach adores his babysitter. Since he's an only child, I'm happy that he can learn to interact with his peers at this young age as he would be learning with a sibling.

Superwoman I'm not. But I do know that if you feel strongly about working full time or if you need to work full time for financial reasons, it can work. And it can work well. Don't be afraid to try it. Your commitment and love for your child should not be questioned.

—TWILA BENNETT, MOTHER OF ZACH, 4

Why I Decided to Work Part Time

This week, as I was walking with my two youngest daughters on the campus of the college where I am an adjunct instructor, a young man on the

(continued on next page)

path caught my attention and reminded me that he had been a student in one of my classes his freshman year. Now a junior, he shared that the course had influenced him in an important way and that he had frequently reflected upon its content over the past two years.

Recently my six-year-old daughter raced into my home office where I was grading papers and announced that she had prepared a surprise for me from the kitchen. As I entered the kitchen, I saw a tray carefully arranged with a glass of juice, a cookie, and a note that read, "Mom, I need you to live."

Frederick Buechner says, "The place God calls you to is the place where your deep gladness and the world's deep hunger meet." The moment with the young man on the path and the moment with my daughter were moments where their hunger and my gladness intersected. Those moments remind me why I have made the choices I have.

My husband and I made two decisions regarding our marriage, our children, and our careers. The first is that we attempt to make mutuality a reality in our relationship. The second is that we want to be the primary nurturers of our children. While I am the primary caregiver of our three children in terms of time, we approach parenting as a team effort. Mark is extremely invested in our daughters, and he meets certain of their needs in ways I cannot. Since he is a full-time seminary student, his schedule is often flexible enough to allow him to cultivate intentional daddy-daughter time with our children when I teach.

Mark has always encouraged me to grow in my gifts. Teaching part time has provided an outlet for me to use my gifts while allowing me the flexibility to be available for my daughters. This ability to be with my daughters in the everydayness of life is something that I am extremely fortunate to have, and it is one of the most treasured dimensions of my life.

One disadvantage of this arrangement of mine, however, is that outside of the four to five hours per week of classroom time, I spend at least four evenings a week, after our daughters are in bed, preparing for class and grading papers. This necessary work means less time for connecting with Mark, less time for maintaining friendships, and less down time for me. It requires me to be intentional about scheduling time for all these activities.

How about financial stress? Yes, with two part-time incomes, we encounter it frequently. But we're also growing in the refreshing satisfaction that comes with living a simpler life.

A few discoveries I have made along the way: Flexibility and options are definitely out there; creativity can take you a long way toward finding a situation that suits you and your family; a supportive husband makes all the difference; balancing your priorities and a constant eye toward discerning the needs of your family will keep you grounded.

—DEONE QUIST, MOTHER OF ELLE, 8, MORGAN, 6, AND ANNA, 3

Why I Decided to Stay Home

I was gazing into the pantry trying to come up with something brilliant for dinner that night. I couldn't keep my mind from wondering what it would be like when I would have to go back to work in a few weeks. It was week six of my eight-week maternity leave. The knot in my stomach and buzz in my head would not go away. All I could think about was how much I did *not* want to go back to work. Don't get me wrong: I loved my job. I had always thought I would definitely return to work, but all of a sudden I was dreading going back. I had spent years at college getting myself ready for my vocation. Even while pregnant I scouted doctorate programs that would move me further along this professional path. But here I was, standing in front of my pantry trying to squelch this feeling that taking care of the child who was quietly napping in her crib was already more fulfilling than anything else had ever been.

Suddenly, I didn't recognize myself. But one thought kept coming into my mind: When is it going to end? When is this wonderful way of life,

(continued on next page)

this time of singing to and feeding and resting next to and bathing and playing with this beautiful little person, going to end? I seemed to fit into this motherhood role perfectly, even though I wasn't very good at it yet. Still, I loved being a mom, and I didn't want it to end! Yet, I hadn't expected to feel this way. This new role in my life came with so many unexpected emotions and realizations.

I'll tell you the truth: I kind of panicked. Playing with the idea of staying home with my child made me wonder what the people in my life would think. I remembered chastising my sister and calling her a Donna Reed wannabe when she told me that her sole purpose in life was going to be finding a husband, making babies, and staying at home with them. I had been one of those people who had questioned what women who stay home with their kids do all day. I remembered the countless policy meetings I had been involved with at the university. I had touted some pretty extreme, liberal-feminist views: Now what would those women think of my desires to quit my job and stay at home with my child? I thought of my husband. Would he feel scared and worried about carrying the financial load on his own? Would he be disappointed in this sudden change in my outlook about what was important and what was valuable in my life? I managed to keep my concerns to myself, not sure if these thoughts were a product of the postpartum hormone fluctuations or if they were really valid.

My first day back at work came with a lot of anxiety, to say the least. That first night my husband returned home moments after I had. I met him at the door and started to cry. I confessed my desire never to go back to work and to stay at home with our little one and her future brothers or sisters. He was surprised but not disappointed. He had actually been wondering how to tell me that he would also like it if one of us stayed home with our children during their developmental years! That night we sat down together and mapped out what our life would be like if I did not go back to work. We decided that we were willing to make significant sacrifices and lifestyle changes in order to make my staying at home a reality.

I never went back to work after that first day. I stayed on-call for a period while the people I worked for found a replacement. The responses to my decision to stay home have been varied. But my family has never gone hungry or unclothed or without shelter. For our family, it has made a lot of sense having a mom at home and a dad in the working world. It has not always been easy, but it has not always been hard either. I truly feel a strong sense of accomplishment and joy with my current lifestyle. I feel as if I have found my niche in life, and I have never grown weary or questioned my decision to stay at home with my children.

A pregnant friend told me that she had always dreamed of staying home with her children, but she didn't see how they could make that work because of their financial obligations. She asked me how my husband and I did it. After some thought, I told her simply, "Where there is a will, there is a way." Ultimately, despite countless details and examples and experiences I could have given her, that is why it works for us. We stay focused on our values, what we think is important, and somehow that has carried us through all our challenges and has enriched all our tribulations.

—BECKY MALMQUIST, MOTHER OF CHLOE, 6, AND KRISTER, 3

What to Do This Month

☐ Find a pediatrician. Most new parents first check to see
which physicians are covered by their insurance carrier and
go from there. Ask around for recommendations. (I found
the most revered and much adored Dr. Addy—a VIP in our
household—this way, and I still thank my friend for the
referral!) You can also call a physician referral service. When
evaluating a pediatrician, consider the following factors: Is
the pediatrician in a practice with others? If not, who covers
for her when she's not available? How can the doctor be
reached in an emergency? Is the office in a convenient location? (You're not going to want to drive to the ends of the
earth when Baby comes down with croup, trust me.)

☐ Think about whether or not you will want a diaper service.
Ask around and do some comparative pricing. If you decide
to go for it, sign up now.

☐ Sit down with your mate and have a heart-to-heart about
the whole working issue. If you are wavering between keeping your job and quitting to stay home, use a solid financial
resource (see Reads of the Month in this chapter) and put
everything down on paper: how much you both make now,
what your expenses are now, how much babies cost, how
you could possibly cut back, how much daycare costs in your
area. Write out a real budget, using your checkbook and
Visa receipts for the last three months to find your actual
needed capital. Then subtract your salary and see what

can/would have to go. Consider extra-income opportunities and at-home businesses (such as Tupperware, Creative Memories, freelance editing, or watching other children) that might make up the deficit and allow you to set your own work schedule. (Note that these businesses will have to be up and running for a year before you make much cashola.) Design a customized plan that will work for you, your husband, and the baby.

❏ Make arrangements for who will care for your other children (and pets!) while you are at the hospital.

❏ Take Fido and Felix to the vet for their annual once-over. Believe me, once the baby comes, your beloved pet slides *way* down your priority list. I have yet to meet anyone who says they still doted on and pampered their pet the same way after they had kids.

❏ Journal idea: Use your narcoleptic hours to write. Tell Baby how silly you felt wearing her dad's "Real Men Fish" T-shirt. Describe your favorite maternity clothes. Fill your child in on how you made the decision to work or not.

Dear Phoebe or Ezra,

It's astonishing to me how much you move. In church the other day, you distracted Daddy from listening to the sermon, he was so captivated by your in utero dance session. Alanna, your second cousin Max's mommy, remembers thinking her baby's movements were like the northern lights moving across the sky, back and forth, changing shape with every flicker. She should know about northern lights, living up there in the Arctic! (You'll know by now that your mother is incredibly proud of being from Winnipeg, the COLDEST CITY IN THE WORLD!) I hope you will inherit my love for winter and, with it, a thickness of blood and hardiness of spirit!

I have to admit, though, it's been a hard few weeks here. Between the pain of all this extra weight sitting on my old broken pelvis, my efforts to be interactive with your brother despite being exhausted again, and those pesky last-month worries, I have been feeling as if Christmas Day will never come. I have started to think a lot about what you might be like, and I've been kind of fearful for some reason. What if you have an illness or a terrible birth defect that will make people stare at you? It would break my heart to see you suffer.

I know there are no guarantees you'll be perfect, but one thing I'm confident is an ironclad fact: No matter what happens in this life, whether it be in your first few months or later, we love you and will stand by you. And Jesus knows how your life will unfold, too. I've got to remember that and quit trying to worry everything until it's okay. He'll see us through, just as He always does.

Anyway, Baby, sorry for the gloomy letter. I do adore you because you're my very own.

Love,
Mama

Stress, Strength, and Sibling Revelry

I created you and have cared for you since before you were born. I will be your God throughout your lifetime.... I made you, and I will care for you. I will carry you along.

—ISAIAH 46:3-4, NLT

Snapshot! All your baby's major systems are working overtime, trying to complete their development before the uterus starts contracting strongly and routinely enough to push her into the outside world. She is working it in there, tensing her biceps, quads, and other muscles, blinking her eyes, swallowing amniotic fluid, and testing her lungs. Even her hiccups are getting her ready to breathe. Last month she trained her senses to hear, taste, feel, and smell. This month, as she heads into the homestretch and the birth canal, she is practicing the skills she will need to thrive after birth, skills like coordination, thumbsucking for soothing, dreaming, and even crying.

Panic-Proof Your Pregnancy

It was one of those phone calls you never forget. A partner in my doctor's practice was on the other end of the line, calmly informing me that my alpha-fetoprotein (AFP) test had showed an increased possibility of my baby's having an open spinal defect. I thanked him for calling, hung up, and burst into tears. Thank goodness Doyle happened to be nearby, and my mom was only a long-distance phone call away.

Of course, the triple test, as it's sometimes called, merely indicated a slightly higher chance that Jonah would have spina bifida, upping the odds from one in 1000 to one in 200. Nonetheless, a stone cold fear settled in my soul, a dread that didn't dissolve until a specialized ultrasound showed that our baby's spine was closed. And even after we had been amply reassured, worries lingered:

- What if the test is wrong, and our baby really does have spina bifida?
- Elizabeth's baby had Down's syndrome, and they had no idea until she was born.
- Could we handle it if this baby had some kind of horrible, disfiguring birthmark?

And, worst of all, sneaky apprehensions lurked beneath the surface:

- What if the unthinkable happened, and Jonah was stillborn?

It does happen, after all.

Suzanna grew up in a family with two brothers who were mentally retarded. You would think she would be anxious about, even obsessed with, the possibility of her own baby having a disability, but the opposite was true: "I was obviously more aware of [the reality of retardation], having two brothers who are mentally handicapped, but I can't honestly say I was worried. I felt that if I was called to [care for a special needs child], I could handle it. I worried more about other things." Her son Henry, now eighteen months old, is not mentally disabled.

Because of the atmosphere in which she was raised, Suzanna had faced the actuality of mental disability over and over. She was better equipped than most of us to deal with that possibility.

Even if you feel fairly confident that your baby will be healthy, chances are you harbor anxieties about other aspects of pregnancy, especially the life changes—mostly uncharted territory—that are swiftly approaching.

"Fear is the dark side of pregnancy, clouding the maternal glow of decorating a nursery and opening shower gifts," says writer Paula Spencer. "Fear of genetics gone haywire. Fear that labor and delivery will be agonizing. Fear about the untold ways that having a baby changes one's life."[1]

   Statistics in Our Favor

Despite overwhelming odds in favor of a healthy, robust baby— the March of Dimes says 97 percent of babies born in America today are free of birth defects—most pregnant women worry that their baby might have to contend with some sort of life-threatening illness or struggle with a birth defect, brain damage, or disfigurement.

Some common late-pregnancy fears:

- *Will a baby interfere with my relationships, my work, my life?* Definitely. But trust me, you'll get through. You may resent the baby for the changes he brings to your life—and you won't be the first mommy to feel this way. But if you take it day by day, you will adjust eventually. Pray for grace and wisdom to adapt and grow in your relationships, especially your relationship with your husband.
- *Will I ever get my body back?* You probably will, even if it takes a while. Remember, "nine months up and nine months down." Of course, I took my sweet time and doubled that to eighteen months before I had my pre-baby body back. Most of my pals, though, took much less time and ate much less in the way of hot-fudge sundaes.
- *What if something goes wrong during delivery?* This is always a possibility, but as I said before, chances are fantastic that everything will

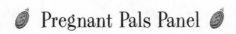

"How Can I Let Go of My Worries and Enjoy This Baby?"

"I feel as if all my friends and my sister have had these textbook-perfect pregnancies and super-healthy babies, too. But for some reason I can't shake the feeling that something might be wrong with my baby. My paranoia wasn't helped by my ultrasound, which showed a possible abnormality in my baby's brain. How can I not become consumed with worry when this baby means the world to me?"

—TENSE IN TORONTO

Dear Tense,

I know firsthand how easy it is to get crazy with worry when it seems like something might be wrong with your precious baby. Hopefully my story will help a little.

Jonathan and I found out on Thanksgiving Day that I was expecting our first child. His brother and sister were visiting and sleeping on the couch—it was 4:30 A.M. I decided to get up and take the test, and *bam!* It was positive, no doubt at all. When I woke up Jonathan and broke the news, we were both elated.

My early pregnancy proceeded like a dream. The only problem I had was a bit of nausea when I was working. As an endoscopy nurse, I knew that some people get motion sickness from watching the vibrations on the scoping screen. When I would get sick to my stomach, my coworkers assumed that was why, so I was able to conceal my pregnancy until the right time.

At eighteen weeks, I was visiting my parents and thoroughly enjoying a meal of chicken soup and bread. In the middle of telling my parents I was having heartburn, I passed out. My mom said I was having convulsions, and they were terrified. When I came to, my dad was giving me mouth to mouth.

In the ER, the staff suggested it was not uncommon for pregnant women to faint. As a former neuro nurse, I knew this was probably no cause for worry, although in the back of my mind I was slightly concerned this might be the onset of epilepsy. After a neurological workup soon after, the doctor pronounced me fit as a fiddle. He just wanted to quickly check my CAT scan results and then I could be on my way.

He went into his office and accidentally left the door slightly open. I was stunned to overhear his words into the phone: "I have a twenty-seven-year-old pregnant woman in my office who appears to have a brain tumor."

Shocked, I confronted the doctor as soon as he came out. "Was that me you were talking about?" I asked, even though I knew it was.

He was quick to assure me that, because of the location of the tumor, it was very, very likely benign. But I knew and he knew that of equal importance was the space the tumor was taking up in my brain. It could press on certain areas of the brain and cause all kinds of problems. Brain surgery, he said, was a definite; the question was when. The two least invasive ways of getting at the growth were through my hard palate and through a nostril, which would be enlarged to the size of a quarter.

I was completely broken up, and so was my family. Jonathan cried, my sister cried, my parents cried. We were all very worried I would have to have brain surgery before my baby was born.

But then the most amazing thing happened. I suddenly felt absolutely fine about the tumor. It was as if God laid His hand on me and said, "You are pregnant, remember, and you have to take it easy here. Don't become engulfed in worry." It was a peace like nothing I could have imagined and like no response I would have naturally had to this kind of crisis.

I would soon have to draw on more of God's peace. Three days after I got the news about my brain tumor, I went to my scheduled ultrasound appointment. We heard joyous news that day: We were going to have a girl. Our little girl! We were so excited. But then came a piece of frightening news: Our daughter had a cyst on her brain, the type of cyst often found in Down's syndrome babies.

We were devastated, even more upset than when I had found out about

(continued on next page)

my own brain tumor. Four weeks later, a follow-up ultrasound revealed yet another anomaly: Our little one's heart cartilage was not developing appropriately, another indication of Down's syndrome. We already loved out baby deeply, and we would have loved her the same with or without the defect. But it was still very hard to accept, especially coming right on top of my health crisis.

While the doctors assured us these two discoveries were not definitely indicative of Down's syndrome—in fact, the findings were considered "soft"—they urged us to have an amniocentesis. No way. I was firm on this. An amnio would be invasive, and finding out for sure if our daughter had Down's syndrome was hardly worth the risk. We tried to lay it to rest and enjoy the rest of my pregnancy.

Meanwhile, lots of people were praying. The word of my tumor had spread beyond our family and church, and congregations all over the place were praying. My dad, a college professor, attended a student's wedding and overheard a member of the bridal party talking about a woman with a brain tumor. It turned out the bridesmaid attended my cousin's church in Canada. The whole church was praying for me. An e-mail coalition of thirty to forty college friends and acquaintances all agreed they would shave their heads as a show of support if my head would have to be shaved for surgery. Jonathan was just amazing through everything, totally caring and supportive. We never fought at all during my pregnancy; we just clung to each other and to God.

At thirty-two weeks, an MRI revealed my tumor was a lipoma, a fatty tumor that was completely encapsulated, which meant it didn't have any branches that could embed themselves in dangerous places. The surgery could wait, maybe even until after my childbearing years. It was grand news.

One day before my due date, and following thirty-five hours of labor, I finally pushed my baby out into the world.

"Is she okay?" I asked my doctor, who had been so wonderful through all the ups and downs.

"She is absolutely perfect," she said, smiling at our new little family. And she was.

One thing I continue to marvel at is how God gave us the heads-up about the tumor. That fainting spell I had twenty-two weeks before Sadie's birth turned out to be completely unrelated to the tumor. It was just a harmless nerve overstimulation related to heartburn. We are so grateful to Him for giving us peace and, most of all, for giving us the gift of our beautiful Sadie.

—RACHEL LAUGHLIN, 28, MOTHER OF SADIE RAY, 7 MONTHS

go smoothly. Even if something does go wrong, unless you give birth in a cab (which only happens on television), highly competent care providers can help you deal with the unforeseen.

- *Will I accidentally let something bad happen to my baby?* I don't know you that well, but I think you'll be terrific. I personally was gripped with the fear that I would do something really ditzy—and potentially tragic—like drop the blow dryer in the bathtub or leave poison lying around for my baby to guzzle. So far, despite my proclivity to airheadedness, I have managed to keep my boys out of harm's way. If I can do it, so can you!

- *Will I be out of control during labor?* Writer Kathleen Kelleher comments on this fear in *Baby Talk* magazine. "Pregnant women have months to contemplate, prepare for, and worry about childbirth, and for many, the fear of childbirth takes center stage," she wrote. "External influences don't necessarily help. Movies and television, for example, often portray the birthing mother as a screaming banshee—hardly a comforting or realistic image."[2] If you're afraid you'll turn into some sort of cussing, apoplectic, hollering-blue-murder version of your self, relax. You probably won't. I had some dramatic moments of wrenching groans and forceful moans, but I never actually yelled—I don't think. And I never called my husband anything unkind, although I did suggest, rather violently, that he not touch me during a contraction. Besides, if you do happen to lose it in a big way, you're not going to care then, and you likely won't be too concerned later either.

- *Will I do something unspeakable during delivery to embarrass myself?* I'm not going to lie to you. The bad news is, yes, you could lose bowel control in front of perfect strangers. But the good news is, you will be losing bowel control in front of the *perfect* strangers, health care providers who have seen it all and who will quickly do the cleanup without batting an eye. As my nurse mother says—

and I quote—"If you've seen one bottom, you've seen them all." Somehow, I found this statement oddly comforting in my hour of need. I hope you will too. Plus, in the moment, you won't care anyway.

Reads of the Month

Will you feed on demand or by the clock? Will Baby sleep in your bed or his own crib? *On Becoming Baby Wise* by Gary Ezzo and Robert Bucknam, M.D., outlines the "schedule-your-baby" school of thought, while *Baby and Child Care* by William Sears, M.D., provides basically the opposite view with his "attachment parenting" philosophy.

Now is the time to research both sides and come to a decision about which approach is for you and your family. Of course, if the baby is premature, your plans might change, so keep an open mind.

• *What if I can't figure out what I should do with the baby in the right way and at the right time?* When I was pregnant with Jonah, I worried about my inexperience with tiny babies. I met a brand new mom at the mall who assured me that my "mothering instincts" would take over. Actually, she was only half-right. I read everything I could get my hands on, and I talked to anyone and everyone about my questions, which I think made up for much of the so-called "instincts" I was supposed to have. Sure, I instinctively adored and cherished my baby and wanted to be with him all the time, but I didn't have an innate way of knowing how to care for his umbilical cord or how to figure out if his low-grade fever was something to worry about or not. That's where good baby-care books (see sidebar above) and veteran moms came in mighty handy.

• Second-time moms face a special fear: *How can I possibly love this baby as much as I love my first?* This one was a biggie for me. It didn't seem possible that I could be as crazy about Ezra as I am about Jonah. Sometimes when I looked at Jonah in all his cute, goofy glory, my heart would snag on this disturbing thought: What if I hurt his feelings—he's so tender—by turning the lion's share of my attention over to his helpless sibling? But every friend, relative, and acquaintance I know who has given birth to more than one baby speaks unanimously on this subject, and I have since joined them: It doesn't seem possible, but somehow, when the new baby is in your arms, your capacity for love expands once more. There is more than enough to go around.

While it makes sense to face your fears and think about the ways in which they are probably unfounded, the best thing you can do is hand them over, again and again and again, to your heavenly Father. Ask Him for the strength and discipline to avoid sliding into a rut of fear-filled thoughts and feelings. "Give your entire attention to what God is doing right now, and don't get worked up about what may or may not happen tomorrow. God will help you deal with whatever hard things come up when the time comes" (Matthew 6:34, MSG).

I know how easy it is to slip into a near-panic state about all the things that could possibly go wrong with your baby, during labor, and postpartum. Cut yourself some slack: Not only are your hormones completely haywire, but you're approaching one of the biggest life changes ever. You're bound to be a little on edge, if not downright loopy! But remember, you are your heavenly Father's beloved daughter, and "God hath not given us the spirit of fear; but of power, and of love, and of a sound mind" (2 Timothy 1:7, KJV).

Alice Chapin, in her book *Nine Months and Counting*, suggests pregnant women fill their minds with the assurance that God is in control: "Today I will remember that it is OK to feel God's relaxation and peace even if there are lots of problems everywhere. It is OK to breathe deeply and feel serene, then breathe deeply again and gain more serenity. Peace is for everyone. God never meant for me to feel anxious or down so much of the time. Imagine God walking beside you (and your baby), holding your hand all day long."[3]

Grand advice. Yes, there are a million and one things to fret about. But don't let fear keep you from enjoying this miracle going on inside your body. What a stunning gift! Instead, claim the peace that is your birthright as a child of God. Claim it over and over until you—and I—get it through our thick skulls that nothing whatsoever is going to happen that we and our Father can't deal with together.

"Don't fret or worry. Instead of worrying, pray. Let petitions and praises shape your worries into prayers, letting God know your concerns. Before you know it, a sense of God's wholeness, everything coming together for good, will come and settle you down. It's wonderful what happens when Christ displaces worry at the center of your life." (Philippians 4:6-7, MSG)

Having Seconds? Preparing
Your Firstborn for the Sibling

Joyce Penner suggests that second-time moms and dads do some play-acting with their little one to prepare for Baby's arrival. She suggests acting out the probable scenario-to-come with dolls and possibly a dollhouse, moving the main players—Mommy, Daddy, the child, Baby, and caregivers—from overnight stays to visits at the hospital and so on. This pretending can help prepare the older sibling and enable her to identify and verbalize her feelings.[4]

I tested this idea with Jonah, and it worked well. A little too well, actually. We were visiting "Grandma Pat" and "Grandpa George" (my dear friend's parents and Jonah's surrogate grandparents) when I used some hockey action figures to represent our newly expanding family. (A hugely pregnant hockey player is a bit of a stretch, but for a three-year-old's kaleidoscopic imagination—no sweat.)

I walked Jonah through all the stages. First we would take him to Grandma Pat's. Then he would sleep overnight in Auntie Rachel's bed, and later he would come visit Mommy, Daddy, and the new baby in the hospital. Scrutinizing his chubby little face for signs of stress, I tried to be as gentle and sensitive as I could. Would he be worried or apprehensive about the abstract I had just constructed? Not a chance. As usual, Jonah was having so much fun at his "grandparents'" house he didn't want to leave. In fact, as I was pulling his snow boots on his feet, his eyes got wide. You could see the wheels turning in his keen little cerebrum. With a satisfied grin, as if he had just found the loophole he had been searching for, he suggested, "You go to the hospital *now*, okay, Mommy?" So much for any heartbreak!

In spite of our best parenting efforts, having a second child can be rough on a firstborn, who, until Number Two pranced into his life, had a cartel going on our hugs, free time, and attention. Experts say there is no surefire way to avoid the growing pains that accompany an expanding family. Jealousy, hurt, and confusion for big brother or big sister are almost definitely going to be a byproduct of bringing Baby home. While you can't predict how your toddler will react to a new baby, you can help smooth the transition during pregnancy and after birth.

"The best way to help siblings become best friends is to show them that the newcomer hasn't robbed them of the most precious thing in their world—your time and attention," say Martha Heinemen Pieper, Ph.D., and William Joseph Pieper, M.D., authors of *Smart Love: The Compassionate Alternative to Discipline That Will Make You a Better Parent and Your Child a Better Person.* "While it can feel a bit overwhelming to be indispensable in so many lives, the more you both can give now, the more you will be repaid later by the secure, happy, confident outlook that your love and attention will instill in them."[5]

The Nifty Nine
Ways for Making Number Two's Homecoming
Easier on Number One

1. Take Number One on a Tour
of the Hospital or Birthing Center

Many hospitals now offer sibling classes for new sisters- and brothers-to-be. They'll show your child a room like the one you'll stay in, chat with the munchkin about his or her fears and concerns over the new arrival, and take him or her to visit the nursery to see what a real, live baby looks like.

2. Designate Childcare for Your Hospital Stay
Well Ahead of Your Due Date

Grandmas and grandpas work well, and so do aunts and uncles and close friends—those tight enough with your clan to wipe runny noses if need be, soothe anxieties, and offer lots of TLC. Whomever your child loves and feels abundantly comfortable with—and who lives reasonably nearby—is a good candidate.

Reads of the Month
Sibling Edition

Franklin's Sister by Paulette Bourgeois

Arthur's New Baby Book by Marc Tolon Brown

God Gave Us Two by Lisa Tawn Bergren (my pal!)

3. While You're at the Hospital, Keep Your Child
Updated As Much As Possible on Your Progress
if Your Labor Lingers On

He'll need to be reassured that everything's okay. Of course, exactly how you approach this tip hinges on your child's age.

4. Ease the Big Brother or Sister That First Meeting

(Drumroll) The first encounter between One and Two is momentous, especially if One is old enough to really grasp what's going on. To ease the meeting, which can be clumsy and confusing for children already nervous about the changes this little creature will bring, try these ideas: 1) Turn Baby over to your husband or Grandma or a nurse. Have both arms ready to greet your older child. 2) Give Number One a present from Number Two. 3) Prop a picture of Number One by your bed and make sure he sees it. 4) Alice Chapin proposes this savvy solution: "Present the youngster with her very own easy-to-use camera a few weeks ahead of Baby's arrival. Showing her how to load it and take pictures of the newborn will heighten the excitement."[6] If your bigger One is still too young even for a disposable camera, snap lots of photos of him with the baby.

5. Keep Your Older Child Involved

Older siblings, ages three and up, will probably get the fact that you need to spend a lot of time with the baby. But include your older child by

 Stockpile Inventory!

Ask a pal or a sister to help you figure out exactly what you need in order to properly care for and feed Junior. If you're expecting Number Two, you may need to take a refresher course. Get together with another new mom—find someone who is pretty well-read on all the information out there—and do a baby-supply inventory: what you need, what you have, what you hope to get at the baby shower Aunt Violet is throwing for you. Then grab that new mom and head to Babies "R" Us to register. After your shower, pick up anything else you need. Beware of sticker shock. Depending on how you fare at your shower, this may be a spendy little trip, especially for first-timers. Be prepared to fork it over to the tune of $300.

enlisting help with baths, commissioning him as diaper courier, having him sprinkle on baby powder, and so on. Number One will feel proud of being Mommy's Helper. If Big Brother is only a wee tyke himself, another strategy is called for. "[Eighteen-month-olds] are like newborns in that their sense of security and inner contentment is still entirely dependent on your positive attention. As a result, your eighteen-month-old lacks the emotional reserves to wait with equanimity while you attend to the new baby," the Piepers write. "While you undoubtedly feel burdened right now, if you can find the space to pay attention to your other…children while you are diapering, feeding, or rocking the baby, they will be more likely to take a kindly attitude toward the new arrival."[7]

6. Stock Up on Cheap Little Gifts for One to Open While Two Is Being Feted with Presents

Toddlers are easy to please in terms of gifts. Last year's stash of Christmas presents will testify to this: The pricey educational toy, with brand new batteries inside, is now rotting in the basement, while the $5 plastic action figure is still Jonah's best bet for hours of amusement. So wrap up a bunch of Matchbox cars, packets of stickers, rubber balls, and the like to have on hand. Also, consider letting One open Two's gifts. Baby won't know the difference, and your big kid will feel included.

7. Make Sure Your Older Child Has Lots of Daddy Time

Your guy can make a lasting gift by giving the older child time with him and by caring for the baby while you take your turn.

8. Validate Your Older Child's Emotions

Vicki Lansky, author of *Welcoming Your Second Baby,* says that it's key to acknowledge your older child's negative feelings. Don't tell him it's wrong to feel jealous or angry with the baby. Discuss his feelings instead. For example, say, "You're feeling left out, aren't you?" or "It's hard to suddenly have to share your mom with another child, isn't it?"[8]

9. Keep Things "Small"

Above all, don't go on and on about how "big" your bigger baby is. These kids are pretty sharp, and they'll soon catch on that being big is not all it's cracked up to be. After all, if being "bigger" is such a bonus, why does the baby get all the attention? If you hype up the big talk too much, your potty-trained, bottle-weaned little man will start stealing his sister's pacifier and wanting to wear Huggies once more. Don't panic though, if you see your child regressing. Expect it to some degree, and let him coast until he feels secure enough to be his big boy self again.

What to Do This Month

☐ Along with your husband, take an infant CPR class. You'll probably never have to use it, but being prepared will make you feel calmer and more in control.

☐ Do the Stockpile Inventory with a seasoned mother.

☐ Read up on the pros and cons of scheduling your baby or feeding her on demand. Decide which is for you so you are informed and can be ready to implement your plan right after birth.

☐ Research stem cell cord blood banking and decide if that's for you.

☐ Pack your bags just in case!

☐ Journal idea: Tell Baby all about his big brother or sister.

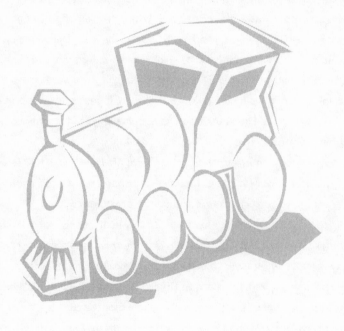

Dear Baby,

You're almost here! Just two weeks left until my due date, Christmas Day. It's actually the middle of the night, and I can't sleep. Apparently neither can you, wiggleworm. Your dad felt my belly the other night and said your movements reminded him of a swimmer doing the breaststroke.

With all the baby stuff piling up in every corner of the house, it seems as if you are really, truly going to be joining us in no time. Daddy's coworkers threw him a surprise baby shower at their weekly meeting, and you got so much pink we went into sugar shock just unwrapping everything. The cake was 70 percent pink and 30 percent blue, which was so clever, but these programmers obviously think there is a 90 percent probability you are female! It's hard not to think of you as being a girl, but don't worry if you're not. I'm bringing a very neutral Winnie the Pooh outfit to the hospital for you to come home in, so no need for embarrassment.

Yesterday was Jonah's birthday party, and after everyone had left—with blue tongues from the whale cake I made—your pop and I talked about how next year we'll have to turn around and party for you, too.

Well, it is 3 A.M., or 4 A.M.—some unearthly hour of the morning anyway. I should make another attempt to sleep or tomorrow will be brutal. I think we are ready for you, so feel free to show up any time. Your room isn't exactly ready—unless you were hoping for an Office Depot motif—but you'll be sleeping in a ruffled bassinet next to me for a couple months anyway. We're not the most organized bunch around here. It's kind of cluttered most of the time, but cozy. Next time I write, I will have held you, rocked you, fed you, and kissed your sweet face. Now that's a beautiful picture.

Goodnight, sweetheart, "'Til we meet tomorrow…"

Love,
Mama

Largess, Lists, and "Love's Labor Done"

Birth
One final push
And you burst forth
Wet and waiting,
Your farewell to the womb
And your welcome to the world.
Love's labor done
I gaze
Awed to silence.
Nine months you've kicked and squirmed
Seen through my womb darkly.
Now face to face
I murmur mother sounds
And touch your cheek and chin.
Love, which bubbled underground
For forty weeks,
Bursts skyward in a geyser
And melts heaven's gates.
In one eternal moment
I hear angel choirs
Echo my alleluia
To your maker and mine.

—CAROL VAN KLOMPENBURG

Snapshot! Your little one is almost ready to meet you, but he's not done growing yet. His head will grow this month in a critical brain-development phase. (Ask your mate to take you out for a nice salmon dinner. Baby needs all the Omega-3 fatty acids he can get for boosted brainpower.) His adorable cheeks are getting chubby due to the fat deposits being added day by day, and all that thumbsucking has toned his sucking muscles. During the last ten days of your pregnancy, Baby will gain half an ounce every day that he stays put in your uterus. If you're lucky, "light-ening" has struck and he has slipped down into position for birth, which means you can breathe again. Hold on—he's almost here!

Feeling "Tremendous"

"When my belly button popped out, I lost it. Belly buttons are supposed to be sweet little dots on your tummy, not actual buttons you push in," writer Jennifer Galvin lamented about that late-pregnancy huge feeling. "Of course, my husband didn't make matters better. He says pregnant women are like turkeys at Thanksgiving: When the timer pops out, they're done. Belly button pops out, baby's done."[1]

Galvin's husband may be right, although the metaphor of plump, but-tery, bursting-at the-seams poultry is somewhat discouraging. Certainly, if my husband called me "Butterball," I would feel justified in impaling him with a meat thermometer.

After about 240 days of gestating, you are probably highly sensitive about the whole issue of feeling large. Big. Colossal. Enormous. Gigantic. Elephantine. Pick your own adjective. (My thesaurus also offered "tremen-dous" as a synonym for the word "huge," which I found quite optimistic.)

Suzanna recalls the emotions that went along with her great, grow-ing girth: "I was getting really sick of getting so big. Not that my doctor thought I was out of control, but I was bigger than I thought I should be. A friend three streets over was three weeks behind me, and she wasn't nearly as large," she says. "My face was big, my legs were fat. When the extra-large stuff from [the maternity store] Motherhood was too small, *that* was really hard."

At thirty-eight and a half weeks, I was so mammoth that only about two articles of clothing in my whole household fit. That included Doyle's camouflage hunting ensemble, which he kindly offered, should I sink that low. One day I had to resort to pulling my brother-in-law's Christmas present out of the bag and wearing it. (That the man received a fleece sweatshirt for Christmas that doubled as a maternity top is a secret between you and me, okay?)

My favorite Big Mama story took place during my first pregnancy. Having interviewed rocker Bryan Adams to preview his upcoming concert in Grand Rapids, I had the opportunity to meet him face to face before his show. But let me just preview this memorable rendezvous with a little history: When I was in junior high and high school, I was a big fan of Bryan Adams. His gritty rock tunes and soulful ballads were the soundtrack of my youth. I only need to hear the first few bars of one of his hits, and I travel back in time to 1984, ghetto blasters, big hair, and first crushes. As an entertainment writer, I've been able to meet lots of musicians, but this encounter was loaded with all the sentimentality, import, and thrills of my best teenage memories.

So there we were, my pal Rachel and I, waiting backstage for The Bryan to emerge. I was highly pregnant at this point and trying not to compare my barrel-like belly with the toned, bare midriffs of the models prancing around. Uh-huh, models. For some reason I can't quite recall (I've apparently blocked it out), there was a bunch of impossibly attractive, statuesque, and fit six-footers sharing the backstage with Rachel and me. It had something to do with them pretending the stage was a catwalk for one of Bryan's tunes. At any rate, they didn't make me feel any smaller.

Then there he was, the rock and roll hero of my youth, grinning widely and coming ever closer. Rachel went catatonic, but in the interests of professionalism, I summoned my powers of speech. "Hi, I'm Lorilee. I interviewed you on the phone the other day," was all I could manage before lapsing into a silly gape. The rocker seemed delighted that I was expecting. He looked me over in the nicest possible way, half-hugged me with one arm, and *pinched my cheek* with his free hand. "Aren't you a little sweetie pie?" he said, referring to my protruding stomach.

It wasn't exactly the stuff adolescent daydreams are made of. In a fantasy, of course, one's pubescent hero would be dazzled by one's sophistication, glamour, and chiseled facial bones, but apparently my chubby cheeks, like Charmin toilet paper, were too much for the guy to resist. Oddly enough, the bigger you get, the more people tend to associate you with those other corpulent, overstuffed cutie patooties—teddy bears—and will pinch and squeeze and pat you accordingly.

The moral of the story is, yes, strangers, kinfolk, and rock legends alike will treat you like an oversized stuffed animal. Smile and endure. It could be worse. They could treat you like that when you're not pregnant.

When in doubt, like the seventh time in one office party someone stares at your belly, bug-eyed, and gasps, "You haven't had that baby *yet?*" cling to this thought: You're not big. You're tremendous.

What to Take to the Hospital

Two or three weeks before your due date, get serious about packing for the hospital. This process is somewhat like packing for vacation only you won't be bringing a two-piece bathing suit or suntan lotion. (In fact, the two-piece should perhaps be put out to pasture. It will no longer serve any meaningful function, except possibly as a dust rag.) You will want to choose items that help you feel comfortable, at home, and equipped for all eventualities, including—and above all—hunger (more on that in a bit).

Pajamas with buttons. Because hospitals offer robes and gowns with the fashion sense of prison uniforms, you may want to bring your own pj's. Not that you will care one way or another about keeping up your sense of style, but you will want to be clean and comfortable. Plus, once you've delivered, you will likely be greeting all kinds of friends and family members, and you'll feel better knowing that your gown isn't flapping open and giving everyone a big show (although—and the cafeteria guy from my hospital can corroborate this—you may not care about modesty either).

Pages for Posterity

If you're a scrapbooker, take along a couple blank pages and a few brightly colored pens so visitors can write their welcome-to-the-world messages for Baby. You'll both treasure forever their words of hope and joy.

Choose dark colors or patterns that won't show stains and look for something with buttons for easy access to your new milking devices. Take a couple of pairs of pajamas because, between sweat and blood and baby pee and who knows what all else, you will long for something clean to change into. When I gave birth to Ezra in December, I only took one pair of pajamas. The result was that my husband had to run around in a blizzard in an effort to find suitable pajamas. It seems that all of mine at home were either flannel (too hot) or shorts sets for summer (too cool). Also, make sure the pajamas are big enough to accommodate your postpartum belly.

Maternity underwear. Yes, maternity. Until your belly—bloated with amniotic fluid, blood, and the like—goes down after a few weeks, you will need all the coverage you can get. Of course, for the first while after you deliver, you won't wear underwear period, although you may have pads stuffed between your legs to absorb all the...er...matter. Another plus to bringing your own: You won't have to wear those bizarre net panties most hospitals issue. And on that note...

Bring your own pads. Seriously, these hospital people are medical professionals who should know better, yet the sanitary pads they hand out are about as useful as stuffing a wad of tissue between your legs. Bring the best pads money can buy, those with high-tech absorption and all kinds of wings, accoutrements, and appendages.

Makeup, soap, shampoo. Showering after giving birth will feel sublime. Using your own shampoo (you won't be, after all, at the Marriott), shower gel, and toothpaste will make you feel human again. Makeup is good for all those inevitable photos taken by visitors. You won't look that great—actually, you'll look awful—but a dash of lip gloss and mascara may make you feel better. Possibly. Well, hopefully.

Reading material. My pal Rachel gave me the best hospital gift: some yummy-smelling shower gel and a couple of glossy magazines. Because I'd had a C-section and would be in the hospital for three-and-a-half days, I appreciated the diversion. This is no time to dazzle the nurses with your literary finesse. Leave *War and Peace* at home and buy something easy-on-the-brain with lots of pictures.

Cameras. Rarely in life will you be as extensively photographed as right after you give birth, just when you are looking so very attractive. But of course it's not all about you—thank goodness. It's about Baby, who will be stunning indeed. With Ezra we went artsy and used black-and-white film. Black-and-white shows Baby's features at their best without all the red blotches and bruises that are sure to show up on that brand-new beautiful face and head. Bring the video camera if you wish to film the event for posterity. (My sister-in-law Tina's labor was filmed, afterbirth and all, by her doting husband, my brother. When they sent the video off to my parents, who were eager to view their new granddaughter, Tina requested that the movie be restricted to immediate in-laws only. She's sensitive that way.)

The contact list. You are not going to feel like digging around your address book for hard-to-read numbers. Make up a master list of the names and phone numbers of everyone you want to call from the hospital. And take your calling card, of course. Some people, myself included, get a real bang out of being called from the hospital rather than being notified secondhand or several days after the birth. Our friends George and Emily are with me on this. They even gave us some incentive to call them when the moment was still fresh: "The sooner the call," they said, "the bigger the gift." Of course they knew before our parents! (The gift? A

hefty gift certificate to a hot tub establishment and a promise to babysit
for the evening—well worth a little hustle on our parts!)

 The Daddy Bag

Your mate should also pack his own bad of essentials, including
a toothbrush, a change of clothes, possibly sweats or lounge
pants in case he sleeps over, magazines, CDs and a player, and
snacks. (Oh, call your husband over here for a sec and tell him I
have something to say: Hey there, Dad! Just between you and
me, it might be a very nice gesture indeed for you to pack a
little token of appreciation for the way your wonderful wife bore
your child. Flowers are sweet, but jewelry lasts longer. A ring or
earrings or a pendant bearing the baby's birthstone would be
just the thing!

Baby stuff. The hospital will have plenty of diapers on hand for your
baby. (Make sure you have plenty of newborn diapers at home, though.)
But Baby will need an adorable "going home outfit." I don't care if the
ultrasound technician bet his left thumb on the fact that your baby was a
girl. He could be wrong, so buy a gender-neutral ensemble. I have heard
more stories of ultrasound readings being incorrect than I care to tell you,
and I'm sure you have too. So pick something perfectly sweet and precious and fabulous—and make sure it's easy to put on. With your limited
experience in dressing a floppy newborn, the last thing you want is an outfit with complicated snaps and flaps, too-small armholes, weird necklines,
and socks that keep coming off. Take a soft, fuzzy blanket to wrap around
your baby and a lightweight knit cap (newborns lose heat out of the top of
their tiny heads). Also, most hospitals now require you to bring a standard,
up-to-code car seat to transport the wee prince or princess home in. (If
they don't, bring one anyway.) If you can, borrow one of those C-shaped
infant neck pillows to support your baby's wobbly neck and heavy little

head. Don't buy one if you can help it; you probably won't use it for more than a month. Obviously, if your progeny will be a winter baby, bring the woolliest, puffiest, coziest baby outerwear you can find. This way you won't have to concern yourself with the prospect of baby getting frostbite, thus reducing your "things to worry about list" from seventy-nine to seventy-eight items. (Oops. Scratch that. You'll have to add "Baby might become so hot and sweaty in the saunalike environment of his pint-sized polar parka that he loses several ounces" to the list, thereby bringing it back up to seventy-nine.) And last but not least...

Food, glorious food. If you end up having a vaginal birth, you'll be able to scarf down a pizza and a pan of brownies if you feel like it. We C-section gals, however, are not so lucky. I was told not to eat a blessed thing after midnight the day before my scheduled surgery. For the first few hours after my C-section, food was the last thing on my mind. But by dinnertime, I was ready for something more substantial than broth, tea, and Jell-O. Placed on a restricted, clear-liquid diet, I had my choice of beef or chicken broth and orange or cherry Jell-O. I tell you, a cube of Jell-O evaporates fast. I tried to keep in mind that there was in fact a good reason for the low-key foods: Apparently introducing anything too sophisticated into my digestive system would have resulted in serious gas pain and pressure. But still, I was soon hungry enough to gnaw on just about anything set before me. Unfortunately, my brother and sister-in-law had no knowledge of my eating regime and arrived bearing edible gifts. "We brought treats!" my brother exclaimed happily, pulling all manner of Christmas cookies, squares, and brownies from his bag. (Suddenly, the tennis ball I had brought because the childbirth class instructor recommended it transformed from back-rub device to weapon. I missed his right temple, although the shock of it all caused him to stop eating for a good forty-five seconds.) So, if you anticipate having a vaginal delivery, bring munchies to the hospital, especially for evening snacks. Cafeterias tend to close early, and nurses have better things to do than to visit the vending machines for you.

Gina's Adventures in Nesting

During my first pregnancy, we lived on the main floor of a 1920s bungalow in Northern Virginia. It was a rental, and our landlord was very cheap. During my first trimester, our sewage system backed up and filled our bathtub with raw sewage. We called the landlord, and she sent her plumber—the cheapest around I'm sure. The plumber decided that he would drain the tub onto the basement floor, which was dirt/cement and, by the way, was home for the washer and dryer, so we went down there often. I definitely wasn't about to take a sweet, new baby into a contaminated (and maybe rightfully condemned) home. So after the sewage dried, I covered the entire basement with lime, and swept it all up with a broom and dustpan. Gross!

During my second pregnancy, I did more normal nesting things: cleaning, laundering the baby's clothes, organizing closets and the attic, buying next season's clothes for our toddler, having a garage sale, and so on. But there were three major projects I insisted we complete before Willa was born: having the kitchen floor stripped and waxed, getting new shelving for the laundry room, and buying a shed for our yard. My husband did not immediately see the connection to a new baby. But this time we lived in a different home; this one we own. The kitchen floor was beyond Mop & Glo, and I needed to have a clean floor for our new baby to crawl on. (Never mind that it would be months before we got to crawling.) The laundry room, right off the kitchen, needed new shelving because I was going to use the dryer as a diaper changing station, so I needed room for diapers, onesies, wipes, clothes, and so on. And we had to have a shed to get all the junk out of the house. I mean, a shed and a new baby—it made perfect sense to me!

—Gina Vos Stansell, 28,
mother of Bendert, 2, and Willa, 5 months

Thinking About the C-Word

In between frantic nesting seizures like regrouting the tub or polishing the miniblinds with a Q-tip, you may want to think about some of your expectations for the birth experience. If you're anything like me, you may be totally unprepared for the possibility of having a C-section. I had this notion that my birth experience would be like that of my female relatives: a relatively quick process ranging in time from two to eight hours. Not that I had anything against a C-section, but I just was so positive it wouldn't happen to me that I even tuned out the birthing class instructor during her brief cesarean speech. But twenty-four hours after my painful contractions started, I was almost at the point of begging for one. When Jonah's heart rate dropped into the fifties and they decided on a quick C-section, I was more than happy to go along with any plan which would result in a delivery.

 Wonder Drug

In a BabyCenter.com poll, 61 percent of new moms had an epidural administered during labor, and 39 percent went drug-free. Of the group that had epidurals, only 19 percent wish they had been able to have a natural birth, while 81 percent expressed no regrets.

I can't say I was too disappointed either. A healthy baby is the same wonderful gift either way. For my second baby, after months of debating, I finally opted to go with a scheduled C-section. It was a hard decision. I felt this would be my last birth experience, and I didn't want to be cheated out of the whole "normal" delivery, the baby's head crowning, the triumphant moment of delivery. I lost track of people who threw in their two bits about why I should push for—nay, *fight*—for a vaginal birth after cesarean (VBAC). Even telling some folks why my doctor and I finally decided on another C-section (because of possible scar tissue from a pelvis I had cracked four years earlier) didn't dissuade them. I finally had to resort to telling people my hips were simply too slim to deliver a baby through the birth canal. (This speech was more effective when delivered over the phone.)

At any rate, I have made my peace with the C-section route, and perhaps you should too, just in case. After all, one out of five births is a C-section.

There's a Sucker Born Every Day

Here's another thing I wish I had known before giving birth: breastfeeding is difficult and stressful—at first. If you choose to nurse, you may expect it to be the most natural thing in the world, but this ultra-natural process takes time and practice to learn. The nurses will probably try to get your little one latched on as quickly as possible to let the bonding begin.

 Formula Works Too

For one reason or another, many of you will choose to bottlefeed. When someone tries to make you feel guilty for this decision, remember that millions of babies have thrived on formula, and chances are great yours will too.

When they brought Jonah to my breast and he began to suck greedily, the nurse was delighted. "He's a good little sucker!" she exclaimed. *Well, why wouldn't he be?* I thought. Little did I know… Over the next few days, I would find out the hard way—by trial and error—just how complicated nursing can be. Newborns fresh out of the hatch tend to sleep constantly, so just as you get the baby latched on—no small feat—the little darling will conk out and slide right off into dreamland. Also, the positioning seems so awkward at first, and it's tempting to hunch forward, tense up,

and generally mess up the whole thing. I was such a hard case when it came
to nursing that a whole battalion of lactation consultants were brought in
to advise, roll towels, arrange pillows, and smash Jonah's face into my
breast. ("Face full of boob! Face full of boob!" one rather kamikaze lacto-
maniac bellowed.)

All that to say, breastfeeding is harder than it looks. But hang in there
for as long as you can. Even just a few tiny teaspoons of colostrom (the
sweet liquid your baby will nosh on before your milk comes in, usually at
three days after birth) will provide him with amazing immunity. Don't give
up just because you think the baby isn't getting enough, but ASK YOUR
DOCTOR OR NURSE FOR THEIR OPINION IF YOU THINK YOU HAVE
REASON TO WORRY! Those wee ones need very little food at first, and
they'll eat when they are hungry. Experts say—and I agree—that after a
few weeks nursing will be second nature.

Cry the Blues, Baby

If you thought pregnancy made you a little teary, just wait until Hurricane
Hormona hits you postpartum. "The day your milk comes in," Alice the
lactation consultant told me, "you will cry at the drop of a hat." Boy, was
she right! As I packed to go home from the hospital, my chest suddenly a
vending machine for my baby's favorite food, I was a soggy mess. The best
advice I ever heard on the matter from anyone (a delivery nurse) was this:
CRY WHENEVER YOU FEEL LIKE IT FOR AS LONG AS YOU WANT. This
is no time to be stoic, what with your hormones causing a deluge of tears.
So just go ahead and cry it out. You can't help these so-called baby blues,
and a good bawl will make you feel better.

If after two or three weeks, though, you still feel weepy and sad, what
you're feeling is not baby blues anymore. Then what you're experiencing is
postpartum depression. Your doctor can prescribe an antidepressant that
will have you feeling more like yourself within a couple of weeks. (Please
see the epilogue.)

A Tale of Two L&Ds

I don't know about you, but I find birth stories to be most absorbing, especially when I'm about to go through it myself. Here are two "Goldilocks" labor sagas—not too scary, not too easy, just about right—for your reading interest. In order for you to get a feel for both scenarios, one is a C-section story and the other, an account of a vaginal birth, pushing, and the whole nine yards. Incidentally, my brother (you remember Uncle Dan and Aunt Tina?) authored the second story, "Zoe's Birthday," in order to document for posterity the miraculous birth of his first child, my niece. (Also, I made him do it.)

Brendan's Birthday (Retold as a Letter to Brendan)

I woke up on the morning of September 30, 1998, with a terrible backache. My abdomen hurt a little, and I was feeling a cold sweat, but my back was absolutely killing me. Because I was still five-and-a-half weeks from my due date, I was planning to go to work—I certainly didn't think I was in labor. I called your Grandma Sommer to tell her how I felt. She said I probably had the flu. But at 9:25 A.M., when I called Dr. Elderkin's office, she suggested I go to OB triage at the hospital. "Better to be safe than sorry," she said.

  **The Truth about
Your Water Breaking**

Chances are you won't have one of those gullywasher experiences in Wal-Mart. Membranes actually rupture in fewer than 15 percent of pregnancies.

I grabbed a fruit bar and a book and headed out the door. When I arrived at the triage area, they hooked me up to two monitors, one for your heartbeat and the other for contractions. The resident doctor checked to

see if I was dilated, but I was not. For about three hours, I just lay in the
bed in pain. They had put in an IV to keep me hydrated and continued to
check on me, but I had no idea what was going on. I paged your daddy at
1 P.M. and told him I was in the hospital but didn't really know anything
at that point. He was concerned, but I told him not to worry.

When Dr. Elderkin came in and checked on me, she said I was having
contractions every one to two minutes! I really didn't even know. The bad

 Pain Management 101

Labor is no picnic. If it were, they would call it "picnic." With my
first baby, I was actually shocked by the intensity of the pain. Some of
my friends didn't seem to think it was all that heinous, but they must
have higher pain thresholds than I. I'm telling you, it can be ferocious.
There is no way to predict or imagine the sensation of your own
labor pain, so you'll just have to brace yourself. You could plan for
drugs, or, if you are the rough-and-tumble sort, you could plan for no
drugs. Pain medications typically fall into two categories:

- *Demerol and other "systemic" meds.* These are supposed to
  "relax" you, which is one way of saying they conk you out
  and hopefully take the edge off. You may get dizzy, drowsy,
  nauseated—or all of the above. I'm not a fan (with my first
  labor it seemed like all this drug did was make me woozy and
  out of it when I needed to be sharp; plus, it hardly touched the
  pain), but some laborers think it helps. Apparently this type of
  drug may make your baby sleepier, but since newborns sleep
  like coma victims anyway, I fail to see the problem there.

- *An epidural block.* An epidural will cut down pain in a specific
  part of your body. It allows you to stay alert during your labor

news was that your heartbeat was not responding properly to the contractions; it was staying steady with the contractions and decelerating
afterwards. Dr. Elderkin told me they would keep me overnight for observation, just to make sure everything was okay.

Daddy showed up at 5:15. They had just transferred me to a regular
birthing room and reattached me to monitors. When the nurse anesthetist
started discussing pain management with me, I thought it was strange
since no one had said I was definitely in labor!

without feeling the big ouch, and it doesn't directly affect
Baby. Oh, it's hard to sit still for five minutes while the anesthesiologist injects the needle into your spine, especially when
you'd prefer to be thrashing about like a wild creature. And
sometimes it doesn't go into the exact right spot, thus failing
to work properly. Also, don't wait too long to ask for it. If
your labor has advanced to a certain degree, your medical
team won't want to impede progress.

Two more things to keep in mind: Don't assume you
can automatically get an epidural if you suddenly can't
handle the pain anymore (ask your doc for more details).
And finally, you might have to wait if the anesthesiologist is
busy. When I went into labor with Jonah, it took me twenty-
four hours to dilate to four centimeters, the magic number
for getting an epidural. But I tell you, once the relief seeped
into my body, I could have—and would have—kissed the
dear, darling, adorable, sweet anesthesiologist. At that
moment I loved him more than any person on the planet.
In fact, two years later, when I spotted that wonderful man at
a play, I had to restrain myself from running up and embrac-
ing him.

Dr. Elderkin came in at 5:30 and looked at the fetal monitor strip. "I just don't like the way this looks," she said. "Since you're thirty-four weeks along, we don't need to worry about fetal development. I think we need to get that baby out of there." I remember looking at the ceiling, thinking they were going to induce labor. Then it hit me. "Does this mean I am going to have a C-section?" She said "Yes." The look of terror and shock on your daddy's face scared me. My eyes started to well up with tears. We were not ready for you to be born yet! The nurse leaned over me and said, "It's going to get really crazy in this room for the next few minutes. Don't be scared. We'll take good care of you and the baby."

Well, she was right. People started running around, throwing gowns on each other. Daddy grabbed the cell phone and called Grandma Sommer. She said Grandpa had just gone to bed, but she would wake him and they would come as soon as possible. He also called your Grandma Walker. Approximately seven minutes after Dr. Elderkin announced she wanted you out, they were wheeling me into the operating room. Everything happened so fast. They quickly put an epidural in my back so I would have no pain. I was numb almost immediately.

Daddy was brought in, and he sat down by my head. I was in the middle of telling him to get me a Kleenex to wipe the tears off my face—so they wouldn't drip in my ears—when Dr. Elderkin commented that the baby had a lot of hair. I said to Daddy, "They cut me already?" I had no idea. At 5:55 we were told we had a beautiful baby boy. What wonderful words.

They asked what your name was, and we said "Brendan." We hadn't decided on a middle name yet. We were still wavering between "Todd" (after Daddy's best friend) and "William" (after my Opa). Daddy wasn't too keen on William, but when I mentioned that half my uterus was lying on the table, he quickly conceded.

You weren't exactly doing great at that point. Your first Apgar score at one minute was three out of a possible ten. That's not good at all. It seems you were having difficulty breathing. Your second Apgar score, at five minutes, went up to eight, which was a lot better. But you were still in some danger, so they quickly showed you to us and then took you down to neonatal intensive care.

The doctors sewed me up and took me into recovery. It was a strange feeling knowing that you had been born, but I hadn't held you or kissed you. After about two hours in recovery, we went down to see you. Grandma and Grandpa Walker had arrived, so they went down with us. You were in an oxygen hood, but they said you were doing well. No one got to hold you until the next morning, but it was worth the wait.

—CHRIS WALKER, MOTHER OF BRENDAN, 3,

AND BROCK, 9 MONTHS

Zoe's Birthday

I'm not a morning person, especially not at 5:30 A.M., but that was when Tina woke me up to tell me she was going into labor. The date was February 8, 2001. We weren't the least bit surprised, considering she was already three days late. Her contractions had begun at 3:30, she said, and now they were regular, about six or seven minutes apart. Our doctor, Dr. Guerin, had told us to head for the hospital when the contractions were less than five minutes apart, increasing in frequency and intensity, and painful enough to take her breath away. Even though her contractions were light, I took the day off anyway.

The day turned out to be pretty uneventful. We cleaned up around the house and waited. Evening came with still no change in the frequency or intensity of her contractions. We decided not to cancel our regular *Survivor* party that night. Our guests came and watched as "Mad Dog" Marilyn was voted out of the Australian Outback. About an hour after everyone left, Tina's contractions became intense, with only three or four minutes between each one. We both took our showers and packed our bags. By 11:30 P.M., I had begun to panic. Tina was drying her hair, and her contractions would double her over in pain. They were now only two to three minutes apart. I thought that we had waited too long and that she was going to have the baby right there in our bedroom. I began running around the house looking for something to clean, straighten, or carry to the car while yelling at Tina to forget her hair and "GET IN THE CAR!" Tina was calmer than I was, and she finished drying her hair, which gave me time to call both mothers for much-needed prayer and "panic" company.

Once we were in the car and safely on our way to Sparrow Hospital, Tina's contractions mysteriously stopped. What was going on? The weather was bad, and we lived forty minutes from the hospital, so we decided to continue heading downtown anyway. About ten minutes later the contractions started again. We joked on the way to that we would see Tina's mother speeding past us on the way to retrieve her first grandchild. We beat her there, but only by about five minutes.

At the hospital, I was ready to hear that Tina was well on her way to delivery. No such luck. One to two centimeters was the word. But because of the weather and our traveling distance, the nursing staff decided to

 Storkbites, Slime, and Your Sweetie Pie

Here she is: Miss America! (Or Miss Canada, Miss Norway, Miss Guam...) Your newborn baby is breathtakingly beautiful and, if the truth be told, totally bizarre looking too. Expect your darling to look a little like a cross between an alien, a gnome, Jane Curtin's *Saturday Night Live* Conehead, and Aunt Myrtle. Her head may be pointy and her eyes as puffy as a blowfish. Slimy is a definite, before they wipe off all the goop anyway. She probably has a birthmark of some kind too, like a "storkbite," a reddish V-shaped mark usually on the forehead or back of the neck. "Angel kisses" are purple-red splotches that "kiss" her eyelids. More serious marks include port wine stains (think Gorbachev), which affect three in one thousand babies, and strawberry hemangiomas, raised crimson dots that show up in 10 percent of all babies born (and which usually disappear by age ten).

keep us for a few hours of observation. Tina was in a good deal of pain, and the last thing we wanted to do was head back home. So began the long wait for our daughter to arrive.

By 4:30 A.M., Tina finally dilated to between three and four centimeters. She was officially in labor, and we were finally admitted to a labor/delivery room. Our desire was for a natural birth with no medication, so for the next three hours my job was to help keep Tina's mind off the pain.

Dr. Kelly, one of Dr. Guerin's partners, came in to check on Tina at about 7:30 A.M. Her cervix wasn't being cooperative and was still only dilated to about four centimeters. After discussing our options, we decided to allow Dr. Kelly to break Tina's water and see if that helped speed things up. After the procedure, Tina's pain became almost unbearable. It made no sense for us to continue without giving her something to help take away the pain. Tina had been in labor for over twenty-eight hours, and considering how things were going, it could still take another twenty-eight. At least with an epidural she would remain comfortable, and we could get some rest and enjoy what remained of the labor experience. The anesthesiologist was wonderful and walked us through the whole process. Tina is deathly afraid of needles, so I was happy she wasn't able to see the one that administers the epidural! The rest of the day passed slowly as we slept, watched *The Price Is Right,* and visited with family.

After thirty-eight hours of labor, Tina finally reached the magic ten centimeters and was ready to push. By this time we were both exhausted and ready to see our baby.

A "normal" delivery (once pushing begins) usually takes an hour or two, or so we were told. Kathy, our nurse, was hoping we would deliver in time for her to see the birth before she went off duty at 7:30 P.M. She had been with us since 7:30 A.M. and had been a joy. *No problem,* we thought. Well, 7:30 came and went with still no sign of birth. Tina did great. Anyone who has been in labor for forty hours and can still find energy to push as hard as she did deserves admiration. My job was to coach and hold up one of her legs. Lori, the new nurse, held the other.

Dr. Bishop (another partner) came in occasionally to help and to check on Tina's progress. At 7:50 P.M. she saw the head crowning and decided to stick around. I can't explain my feelings when I finally saw the head crowning. It was the greatest feeling on earth, knowing that our daughter's birth was imminent. During the next few minutes there was a flurry of activity in the room as instruments were set in place and everyone got into position. The anesthesiologist had turned down Tina's epidural a few hours earlier to prevent her from becoming too numb. Apparently she had turned it down too far, and Tina was once again in excruciating pain. I have always heard horror stories of delivering mothers screaming obscenities, grabbing loose flesh, or hurtling nearby objects. Tina, however, was a model patient with only one comment that bears mentioning. Halfway through the pushing process during a particularly painful moment, my wife found the strength to yell, "GET IT OUT OF ME!" Heeding the outburst, Dr. Bishop told me to use the call button to call the anesthesiologist. I balanced on one leg, held one of Tina's legs, and somehow managed to push the call button. Tina received a few local anesthetics to numb the pain just in time for our daughter to be born.

Zoe Marie Sue Reimer came kicking and screaming into the world at 8:09 P.M. on February 9. My first memorable words to Tina when I saw our baby were, "It's a girl, honey. We don't have to redecorate." Through tears, I got to cut the cord and watch as mother and daughter first bonded. Even Kathy peeked in and got to see Zoe before she left. Now it was time for Zoe to get cleaned up, weighed, and measured. Apparently babies do not like being poked and prodded after nine months of seclusion because Zoe voiced her displeasure with enthusiasm. She scored an eight out of ten on the Apgar scale, and her 21-inch body weighed eight pounds, eight ounces. After two hours of recovery and a visit from some very interested family, we were ready to grab some much-needed sleep. Tina and I were now parents, and a whole new adventure had begun.

—DAN REIMER, FATHER OF ZOE, 15 MONTHS

The Nifty Nine Days to Labor:
The Countdown Begins

Of course, everyone's prelude to birth goes a bit differently. But there are enough similarities that your story, and mine, might go a little something like this:

Nine Days

Wake up in a frenzy of nesting. Wash, wipe, sweep, dust, vacuum, and disinfect the house. Mid-morning, because the threat of ring-around-the-collar seems terrifyingly real, sterilize the ironing board. Take inventory of spices and send husband to market for cumin. Account for all rubberized containers you thought you owned; call Tupperware consultant and order missing lids. Plop onto sofa in exhaustion and read an alarming article about the newfound dangers of Scotchgard. Rake at sofa with fingernails, trying

 Braxton Hicks

For months already you may have noticed your abdomen tightening, sort of bunching up for half a minute or a minute. These random, usually painless contractions are called Braxton Hicks, and about now you may think they're a real hassle. Unless you've gone through labor already, it may be really tough to distinguish Braxton Hicks contractions from the real deal. Actual here-we-go contractions are considerably longer, more concentrated, and more painful. Stay in your doc's good graces and don't make him get out of bed at 4 A.M. until your contractions are sixty seconds in duration and five minutes apart. Other signs that your labor pains aren't a false alarm: lower back pain, the shakes, diarrhea, and the advent of blood-streaked mucus.

in vain to remove harmful chemicals. Direct husband to take sofa down to the basement and replace it with the futon from your first apartment.

Eight Days
Tell husband to feel your belly during a contraction and describe the sensation: Bunchy? Hard? How bunchy on a scale of one to ten? How hard? Call sister-in-law and find out just how bunchy and hard her belly got before she determined she was in labor.

Seven Days
Visit ob-gyn and hear the news that you are "fingertip" dilated. Make long-distance phone calls to share the good news with loved ones.

Six Days
Fret about Radon, events in Chechnya, potholes, your gene pool (specifically, Uncle Earl), and much, much more.

Five Days
It's a mere twenty-four hours before your actual due date, and friends, family members, coworkers, and other interested parties begin to ring your phone off the hook. Just as you are about to install caller ID, you sneeze and bodily fluid emerges. Could it be your water breaking or just a sneeze-related incident? Call your doctor and discuss the difference between incontinence and the rupture of amniotic membranes.

Four Days
Husband takes one last stab at persuading you that "Larry" is a suitable baby name. Tell him you'd rather call the kid "Braxton Hicks."

Three Days
Call Best Girlfriend to come over immediately. Page your husband at work: There's something in the toilet that looks like it could be a mucus

plug. The three of you put your heads together (literally) and gaze for a time at the object. Determine that, yes, it could be nothing else but bloody show!

Two Days

Run three stop signs and arrive breathlessly at the emergency room. Excitedly tell the receptionist that your contractions are five minutes apart! Double over in pain and try to speak through contractions. Unpleasant nurse confirms Paranoid Thought #37: Since you are only one centimeter dilated, you will not be admitted to the hospital and must return home. She advises you to "get a grip," and you somehow restrain yourself from gripping her around the neck.

One Day

Contractions have gone way beyond bunchy or not bunchy. You can talk through them all right—as long as you're yelling! Determine that the hospital *will* keep you or else a hostage situation might well develop. During a short but sweet pain-free interval, bid a teary farewell to the cat. Tell him to hold down the fort—it's time!

"Love's Labor Done"

For several weeks before my due date, I experienced Braxton Hicks contractions. Having gone through labor once before, I knew it would hurt like crazy when the real thing was upon us. Of course, what if this time my labor progressed entirely differently and I delivered fast, with no warning, on the laundry room floor? One more thing to be paranoid about.

Because dear Dr. Grey and I had concluded months beforehand that a C-section was the way to go, all I had to do was show up on the appointed date and time and have the nice medical professionals extract child Number Two. I missed the drama of waiting and wondering when my baby's birthday would be. Then I remembered the pain of labor, and drama seemed overrated. Still, it was possible I could go into labor earlier than the date of my scheduled surgery. This very thing had recently happened to my friend Heather.

Doyle could not wait to see my internal organs again. Some husbands shudder at the thought of their precious wives going under the knife. Not Doyle; it's all the Discovery Channel for him. "They are now making the cut, hon…cutting, cutting, cutting…It looks like they've got your bladder—or some quivery mass of flesh—outside of you. It's sitting on your stomach! Hey cool!" Last time the docs had to ask him to please step away from my midsection. They were afraid his gum might fall out of his mouth and into my body cavity.

Doyle got his wish.

On the morning of December 19, 2000, we awake to the blare of the alarm at 5 A.M. My surgery is scheduled for 6. We quietly dress, and I put on makeup and do my hair just to have something to do. It is an odd sensation, knowing I will be cut open within a matter of hours. For some reason, I feel a bit frightened.

We drive through the darkness of the cold, wee hours of the morning and arrive at Metropolitan Hospital in five minutes without ever seeing another car. When we get to the hospital, Doyle realizes he forgot the camera. I stay while he races home to get it.

My first nurse is a calm, efficient woman who explains in detail the hospital's policies about liability and that sort of thing. I try to listen, but my thoughts wander. I sign the release forms anyway and change into a green gown. I shove my hair into an attractive plastic surgical cap—thank goodness I had styled it. My apprehension begins to mount as I take in the antiseptic surroundings of the hospital. I pray for courage, for my baby right at that moment, and for a safe delivery. The nurse is wearing a thick silver ring with Hebrew letters on it. I ask her what it means. "I am with you always," she says, quoting Jesus. Peace settles and I am ready.

Doyle returns and changes into blue scrubs. I tell him he looks like

George Clooney. (It's good for some comic relief.) Dr. Grey and I chat as the gurney rolls down the hall.

"Do you know what you're having?" she asks.

"Well, they told us they were 70 percent sure it's a girl."

"Hmmm. Usually they give you a higher percentage, like 90. Seventy is not too high," she says, adding with a grin, "They told me my second son was a girl, too."

 Reads of the Month (and Beyond)

The Baby Book: Everything You Need to Know About Your Baby from Birth to Age 2, by William Sears, M.D., and Martha Sears

Caring for Your Baby and Young Child, Birth to Age 5 by the American Academy of Pediatrics

What to Expect the First Year and *Touchpoints* by T. Berry Brazleton

And my new guide to Baby's first year, due summer 2003. (Okay, so if your due date is earlier than that, keep me in mind for your next.)

For the first time, it occurs to me we could actually be having another boy, despite our strong "feeling" otherwise and the overwhelming majority projection that this is our Phoebe.

At any rate, there is no time to further contemplate this astonishing idea. As I am wheeled into the surgery room, harsh with glaring overhead lights, I wonder why I don't remember it from last time. Probably because I had just endured 24 hours of mind-bending pain. The chipper anesthesiologist arrives with long needles. "Keep your back as straight as possible," he advises. "You'll feel a poke, then some pressure. Just hold very still and this will be just beautiful."

Hello! Ouch! That I can definitely feel. The sensation is sharper and deeper than I remember.

"Perfect! Excellent! This is the best job I've ever done!" The wiry dope doctor is high on his accomplishment. His enthusiasm boosts my spirits.

When they determine I can't feel anything lower than my chest, they hang a curtain a few inches from my face to block my view. Suddenly, doctors and nurses and interns and all kinds of people who seem to be passing surgical instruments to one another surround me. What was that "clink" of metal I just heard? Did someone just say "scalpel"?

I panic. "Where's Doyle?" I ask, needing him beside me in the worst way.

"Get the husband in here," Dr. Grey orders.

Doyle hustles to my side, and we hold hands tightly. He peeks over the curtain, of course, and sees them cut an incision just below my bikini line. This time, he keeps the play-by-play to himself.

I lie there and try to breathe relaxing cleansing breaths. Dr. Grey and two twentysomething residents, Drs. Michelle Becher and Molly O'Kane, engage in girl talk. Michelle is pregnant herself, I learn, and Dr. Grey is planning to adopt a baby from China. *How nice for her,* I think, actually getting into listening to their conversation.

I feel pressure, pulling, and jostling. I know they are pulling the baby out, head first, then one shoulder, twisting, then the other, and finally they yank the whole body into the outside world.

"It's a boy!" Dr. Grey exclaims as boisterous screaming ensues.

My eyes and Doyle's meet, and in one electrifying moment we realize shock so great it's as if someone stuck our fingers in a light socket. A boy! *The pink stuff will be going back to the store,* I think, oddly.

Dr. Grey brings my squalling son up to my face. "Hello, baby. Hello sweetheart." Tears stream down my face. (A boy!)

He is the most gorgeous thing in the world, irate, vociferous, as red as a boiled lobster, and covered in slime. If possible, his howling is even more earsplitting than his big brother's had been three years ago.

"Why is he so red? Is he okay?" I ask anxiously as they carry him off somewhere, out of my view, to be bathed, weighed, measured, and manhandled. I'm dying to hold him. (A boy!)

"Oh yes, the redder the better," a nurse answers. Doyle accompanies his son as he undergoes these first assessments of his young life.

"Seven pounds, 7 ounces, 19.5 inches" is the first of the news. Then the Apgar Score: "Nine point five," I hear someone say. Pride and gratitude swell up inside me. He's so very, gloriously healthy! *Thank You, God.*

"What's his name?" Dr. Grey asks through the curtain that still separates us. She's stapling me shut.

"Ezra," I say, filled with the euphoria reserved for such moments. Throughout my pregnancy, I had told people I actually liked our boy's name better than our girl's name, even though we were sure we were having a girl. I knew then it was true.

A boy! My Ezra.

What to Do This Month

☐ Go have that baby!

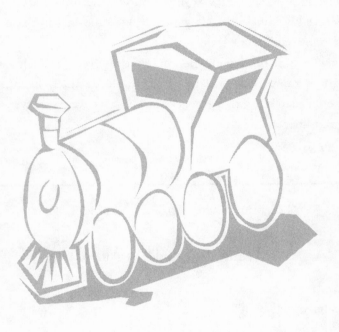

Postpartum Depression
Is No Laughing Matter

Girls, I am begging you, if you think you might have postpartum depression (PPD), please call your doctor to discuss treatment options. I know we have shared some jokes over the last nine months, but on this topic I am dead serious. If it's been more than two or three weeks since you've delivered and you still feel really weepy, sad, and lethargic, you're no longer dealing with baby blues.

Thanks to celebrities such as Marie Osmond, who told the world about her debilitating bout with PPD, the stigma of this chemical imbalance has lifted—somewhat. Nonetheless, I can't tell you how many new moms I've talked to who felt they *did* have postpartum depression but wouldn't accept the help that is available to treat this disorder! This makes me crazy because there is nothing wrong with receiving the treatments that exist—namely medications such as Prozac and Zoloft. Listen to me when I tell you that PPD is nothing you caused or could have prevented. It's *biological*, for Pete's sake, a chemical response to the huge hormonal fluctuations in your body. You can't try and be strong; you can't "outspiritualize" these sad feelings. You can't wait them out. And you sure can't just "snap out of it." This is wrong thinking, girlfriend.

After my second pregnancy, I could not shake the gloominess I felt any more than I could have "gotten over" gestational diabetes or some other pregnancy-related illness. Thank goodness I learned from what my dear mom went through, her six years of almost-crippling clinical depression. I think if I hadn't experienced firsthand the horrific effects of that depression, I, too, may have tried to tough it out. Instead, I went on a low-dosage of Zoloft and, within a couple of weeks, felt the sunshine again, regained my positive outlook, and thanked God for creating this medication through His scientists and researchers!

The best thing you can do if you feel you might have PPD is consult your doctor. In most cases, he or she will write a prescription for you, and you'll be feeling more like yourself in a couple of weeks. If you feel, however, as if your doctor is not taking you seriously, please don't quit until you find one who does. (And, hubby, if your wife doesn't have the strength to take these steps herself, *step in and support her.* Help her get the help she needs.) Do keep in mind that PPD can last up to a year after delivery, so be prepared to commit to staying on medication as long as your doctor thinks necessary. There is so much at stake here—not only your happiness, but your baby's well-being too. Do it for yourself, or do it for your family, but definitely stop this thing in its tracks just as soon as you can.

It's just the smart thing to do.

Notes

Prologue

1. Sherman Silber, M.D., "Getting Pregnant," BabyCenter.com, 2001.

Month One

1. Joyce Penner, *What to Pray When You're Expecting: Hopes, Prayers, and Dreams During Pregnancy—For Mom and the Whole Family* (Ann Arbor, Mich.: Vine, 2000), 57.

Month Two

1. Susan Maushart, *The Mask of Motherhood* (New York: W. W. Norton and Company, 1999), 43.
2. Arlene Eisenberg, Heidi E. Murkoff, and Sandee E. Hathaway, B.S.N., *What to Expect When You're Expecting* (New York: Workman, 1996), 102.
3. Karen Vogel, "The First Trimester," BabyCenter.com, 2000.
4. Karen Vogel, "The First Trimester."
5. Penner, *What to Pray,* 29.
6. Leslie Brandt, *Psalms Now* (St. Louis, Mo.: Concordia, 1973), 51.

Month Three

1. Jean Lush, *Women and Stress* (Grand Rapids, Mich.: Revell, 1992), 113.
2. Jean Lush, *Emotional Phases of a Woman's Life* (Grand Rapids, Mich.: Revell, 1987), 139.

Month Four

1. Nora Ephron, as quoted by Alice Chapman, *Nine Months and Counting: Bible Promises and Bright Ideas for Pregnancy and After* (Wheaton, Ill.: Tyndale, 1999), 8.
2. Vicki Iovine, *The Girlfriend's Guide to Pregnancy: Or Everything Your Doctor Won't Tell You* (New York: Pocket, 1995), 17.
3. Cheryl Richardson, *Take Time for Your Life: A Personal Coach's 7-Step Program for Creating the Life You Want* (New York: Broadway, 1999), 185.

Month Five

1. Keith Bellows, "How to Share in Your Wife's Pregnancy," BabyCenter.com, 1998.

2. Armin A. Brott and Jennifer Ash: *The Expectant Father: Facts, Tips, and Advice for Dads-to-Be* (New York: Abbeville, 1995), 43.

3. *Parents Expecting,* Winter 2001-2002.

4. Dr. Jerrold Shapiro, Ph.D., as quoted by Keith Bellows, "How to Share."

5. Ron Schultz and Sam Schultz, *How to Pamper Your Pregnant Wife* (Minnetonka, Minn.: Meadowbrook, 1996), 47.

6. Celeste Fremon, "One Great Dad: Hockey Legend Wayne Gretzky Builds His Own Team," *Fit Pregnancy,* August/September 2000, 84.

7. Carol Stahmann Dilfer, *Your Baby, Your Body: Fitness During Pregnancy* (New York: Crown, 1977), 2.

8. Dana Sullivan, "Do It Right: Great Upper Body Strengtheners," *Fit Pregnancy,* August/September 2000, 68.

9. Shelly Lavigne, *Boy or Girl? 50 Fun Ways to Find Out* (New York: Dell, 1992), 8, 15, 20.

Month Six

1. Leah Hennen, "Pregnant from Head to Toe," *Baby Talk,* October 2000, 35.

2. Tracie Hotchner, *Pregnancy and Childbirth* (New York: Avon, 1997).

3. Raina M. Paris, *The Mother-to-Be's Dream Book: Understanding the Dreams of Pregnancy* (New York: Warner, 2000), xix.

4. Eisenberg, Murkoff, and Hathaway, *What to Expect,* 223.

5. Patricia Garfield, *Women's Bodies, Women's Dreams* (New York: Ballantine, 1988, 1991).

6. Celeste Fremon, "Star Moms: Show and Tell with Janet Jones Gretzky," *Fit Pregnancy,* August/September 2000, 34.

7. Paris, *Dream Book,* 281.

Month Seven

1. Iovine, *Girlfriend's Guide,* 120.

2. Iovine, *Girlfriend's Guide,* 122.

3. Glynis Costin, "8½ Months & Counting," *In Style,* July 2000, 7:7, 202.

4. Costin, "8½ Months," 202.

5. Jennifer Galvin, "Feeling Whale-ish?" BabyCenter.com, 2000.

Month Eight

1. Paula Spencer, "The Panic Free Pregnancy," *Baby Talk,* November 2000, 75.

2. Kathleen Kelleher, "TBA," *Baby Talk.*

3. Alice Chapin, *Nine Months and Counting: Bible Promises and Bright Ideas for Pregnancy and After* (Wheaton, Ill.: Tyndale, 1999), 80.

4. Penner, *What to Pray,* 143.

5. Martha Heinemen Pieper, Ph.D. and William Joseph Pieper, M.D., *Smart Love: The Compassionate Alternative to Discipline That Will Make You a Better Parent and Your Child a Better Person* (Boston: Harvard Common, 1999).

6. Chapin, *Nine Months,* 19.

7. Pieper and Pieper, *Smart Love.*

8. Vicky Lansky, *Welcoming Your Second Baby* (Minnetonka, Minn.: Book Peddlers, 1995), 66.

Month Nine

1. Galvin, "Whale-ish?"

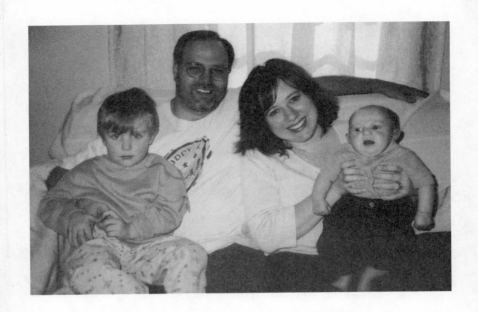

LORILEE CRAKER lives happily in Grand Rapids, Michigan, with three men in various stages of hair loss. Doyle, the patriarch of the Craker family, is now able, due to a swiftly receding hairline, to show off a cool scar from childhood when his big sister belted him with a stick. (Or did he pull a fan down on his head? The details are a little fuzzy.) Jonah, a normally smiley preschooler, but not for his mother's book photo, of course, used to be as bald as a hockey puck. Baby Ezra is so far even more hairless, although, as this book went to print, his mother glowingly reported an adorable tuft sprouting on the west side of his head. Pierre the cat (not pictured) has bragging rights as hairiest Craker man.

You can reach Lorilee by writing to lorilEJ@aol.com, or learn more about her books at her Web site, www.LorileeCraker.com.